"Peter Kevern offers a deeply humane and theologically rich reflection on dementia, urging us to see not just decline but divine presence in the midst of forgetfulness. With wisdom, clarity, and pastoral warmth, he challenges the church to move beyond fear and toward a faith that embraces vulnerability. This book is a gift—an invitation to rethink what it means to be human, to belong, and ultimately, to touch God."

—JOHN SWINTON
Professor in Practical Theology and Pastoral Care, University of Aberdeen

"This is a rich, pastorally sensitive, personally involved, theologically wide-ranging, creative piece of scholarship. I am not sure whether Peter Kevern has given us an academic volume that is unusually engaging and readable or a pastoral and practical book that is unusually academically serious and careful, but either way, it is a valuable contribution."

—KAREN KILBY
Bede Professor of Catholic Theology, University of Durham

"There are three key qualities to this book. The first is that it is grounded in the intimate experience of dementia in a loved one. The text is informed by these experiences, which are handled with extraordinary sensitivity. The reader is taken into the complexity and perplexity of this disease. The second is the way in which *Touching God* is shaped by a generative grasp of the Christian theological tradition. There is wisdom in the exploration of the agency of God in the face of human fragility. The third is the author's ability to ask and hold difficult questions. These chapters touch life, hope, theology, belief, and the very nature of God. Read this—you will not be disappointed."

—JAMES WOODWARD
Principal, Sarum College, Salisbury, United Kingdom

"*Touching God* is a theological journey into the depths of dementia in which Christ is always organically present. It not only offers a transformative vision of living and dying with dementia, but also enriches our understanding of the mystery of the incarnation."

—JOANNA COLLICUTT
Supernumerary Fellow, Harris Manchester College

Touching God

Touching God

Dementia and the Bodies of Christ

PETER KEVERN

CASCADE *Books* · Eugene, Oregon

TOUCHING GOD
Dementia and the Bodies of Christ

Copyright © 2025 Peter Kevern. All rights reserved. Except for brief quotations in critical publications or reviews, no part of this book may be reproduced in any manner without prior written permission from the publisher. Write: Permissions, Wipf and Stock Publishers, 199 W. 8th Ave., Suite 3, Eugene, OR 97401.

Cascade Books
An Imprint of Wipf and Stock Publishers
199 W. 8th Ave., Suite 3
Eugene, OR 97401

www.wipfandstock.com

PAPERBACK ISBN: 979-8-3852-3255-0
HARDCOVER ISBN: 979-8-3852-3256-7
EBOOK ISBN: 979-8-3852-3257-4

Cataloguing-in-Publication data:

Names: Kevern, Peter [author].

Title: Touching God : dementia and the bodies of Christ / Peter Kevern.

Description: Eugene, OR: Cascade Books, 2025 | Includes bibliographical references.

Identifiers: ISBN 979-8-3852-3255-0 (paperback) | ISBN 979-8-3852-3256-7 (hardcover) | ISBN 979-8-3852-3257-4 (ebook)

Subjects: LCSH: Dementia—Religious aspects—Christianity. | Memory—Religious aspects—Christianity. | Dementia—Patients—Religious life. | Pastoral Care.

Classification: BT732.4 K48 2025 (paperback) | BT732.4 (ebook)

VERSION NUMBER 052025

All Scripture quotations, unless otherwise indicated, are taken from the Holy Bible, New International Version®, NIV®. Copyright ©1973, 1978, 1984, 2011 by Biblica, Inc.™ Used by permission of Zondervan. All rights reserved worldwide. www.zondervan.com The "NIV" and "New International Version" are trademarks registered in the United States Patent and Trademark Office by Biblica, Inc.™

To my mother, Daphne. My first and best theological teacher.

Contents

Permissions | IX
Acknowledgments | XI

Introduction: Dementia in "The Bad Home" | 1

1 Why are we so afraid of dementia? | 14

2 What sort of a God is to be found in dementia? | 33

3 Sharing the mind of Christ | 48

4 Symeon of Emesa and the "holy fools" of God | 66

5 "Do you think he has a soul?" Eucharist, *anamnesis*, and the forgetfulness of dementia | 83

6 From cognition, through emotion, into spirit: Continuing faith in the midst of dementia | 100

7 Mum's last day: Does the flesh pray? | 113

8 Touching darkness, touching God: Dementia and the end of all things | 128

Conclusion: Deconstruction incarnate and the Incarnate, deconstructed | 143

Bibliography | 149

Permissions

The extract from "The Long Goodbye" is reproduced with kind permission of the Alzheimer's Society.

The poems "The Bad Home" and "Glimpses" are reproduced by kind permission of John Killick.

Some of the material comprising chapter 1 has appeared in a different form in:

> Peter Kevern. "The Fear of Dementia and the Challenge to Personhood: Exploring the Depths of Our Existential Dread." In *Understanding Existential Health for Dementia Care: Supporting the Bio-Psycho-Social Approach*, edited by Lars Danbolt, Peter La Cour, Tatjana Schnell, and Gry Stålsett. London: Routledge 2025. Copyright (2025) Routledge. Reproduced by permission of Taylor & Francis Group.

Some of the ideas developed in chapters 2, 3, and 4 were previously explored in the following papers:

> Peter Kevern. "The Grace of Foolishness: What Christians with Dementia Can Bring to the Churches." *Practical Theology* 2.2 (2009) 205–18.
>
> ———. "Sharing the Mind of Christ: Preliminary Thoughts on Dementia and the Cross." *New Blackfriars* 91.1034 (2010) 408–22.
>
> ———. "What Sort of a God Is to Be Found in Dementia? A Survey of Theological Responses and an Agenda for Their Development." *Theology* 113.873 (2010) 174–82.

Acknowledgments

THE INSPIRATION BEHIND THIS book is my mother, Daphne Kevern, who died with dementia in 2004. As well as providing the motivation for me to think and write on the subject, she provided me with the tools and the model for how to do it. She encouraged me to ask questions, took them seriously, and gave thoughtful answers to my wild and immature theological speculations.

Others contributed in different ways. My father, through his example of patient love, dogged persistence, and courage in the face of a condition that also took from him and my mother the opportunity to enjoy some of their best years together. Father Pat Kilgarriff, who helped to keep my spiritual life more or less on track during the intense periods of writing and reflection. The colleagues and friends—Edward Tolhurst, Karen Kilby, and John Swinton—without whose comments and guidance this book would have many more shortcomings.

Finally, my wife Rachel, who loved and tolerated me through the many times during the writing of this book when I was absent from her in spirit, bringing me back down to earth and into my body with grace and wisdom. She deserves my gratitude, love, and, perhaps, apologies!

Introduction
Dementia in "The Bad Home"

The Bad Home

God so loved the world
But He did not love this place.
All I want to do is die.
So why can't I be let to do so?
Why can't you just lay down your head?

I walk and walk
But there is no God,
Not in this place.
This is the Bad Home—
He has forgotten its existence.

I get up and walk till I fall.
Sinful though I be
I'll ask God for His mercy.
I'm too old to do anything.
I'm just a dustbin.

. . .

God so loved the world
But He doesn't love me.
I used to be happy,
But now I'm angry with Him
Because I'm still here.[1]

DEMENTIA HAS MANY FACES, and there are many different stories to be told about it. In the first place, there is the clinical story, the bare account of

---

1. Killick and Cordonnier, *Openings*, np.

what it does to the body, and what happens as a result.[2] There is the story of the medical researchers, of a heroic struggle to find a "cure" that will "defeat" dementia once and for all.[3] There is the story told by politicians, planners, and public health officials of a tidal wave of long-term social care needs that threatens to overwhelm our public services and impoverish the nation.[4]

This is not, however, dementia as we experience it, for which the clinical, medical, and policy stories seem too small and too mechanical. The stories we tell among ourselves, of our own dementia or of dementia among those close to us, are more vivid and frightening, rich in metaphors of theft, chaos, betrayal, and "living death." Our stories about people living with dementia are stories of loss, confusion, and sadness: of people eventually failing to recognize those closest to them; and, in turn, becoming unrecognizable as their language, personality, and sense of self-identity all seem progressively to slip away.[5]

Finally, for Christians, there is an additional register in which we may experience dementia: as a potential betrayal of faith. Although, to the eyes of exceptional faith, dementia may seem like a "glorious opportunity" for a deeper discipleship,[6] for most of us dementia challenges our faith, casting us into the "Bad Home" where faith is not, and God appears to have departed. The images of God we have to hand—our supreme Father in heaven, our conversational friend, the one responsive to our needs and returning

---

2. "Dementia is a syndrome that can be caused by a number of diseases which over time destroy nerve cells and damage the brain, typically leading to deterioration in cognitive function (i.e. the ability to process thought) beyond what might be expected from the usual consequences of biological ageing. While consciousness is not affected, the impairment in cognitive function is commonly accompanied, and occasionally preceded, by changes in mood, emotional control, behavior, or motivation." World Health Organization, "Dementia." It is conventional to start a book on dementia with a recitation of facts and figures, but this is both tedious and quickly outdated. For current background information, see the Alzheimer's Society website at https://www.alzheimers.org.uk/.

3. Alzheimer's Research UK, "Rising to the Challenge."

4. Shepheard and Woodrow, "GPs to Bear the Brunt." But see also Wilson, "What Dementia 'Tsunami'?"

5. "We strive, as do millions of others,
to figure out ways to live in the presence of a disease
that mercilessly erases my husband's life
bit by bit, memory by memory.
Some days we manage, some days we don't." Fox, *I Still Do*, 67.

6. Bute and Morse, *Dementia from the Inside*.

Introduction

our love—lack purchase in this place, where it can seem that "God so loved the world but He doesn't love me."

So if the experience of dementia is of the "Bad Home" where there is no God, we need to do two things: first, to reflect on our experience and understanding of dementia as a threat to who we are "before God" and, second, to ask about what sort of God is, nevertheless, to be encountered there. That is, we need to develop a specifically *contextual* theology, one that, while it reflects on what our theology might have to say about dementia, makes a point also of exploring what our experience of dementia means for our theology.[7] It needs to ask, "What does God (or the Christian tradition) say about dementia?" and also, "What does the fact or experience of dementia say about God?" These are the underlying questions driving the present book.

My reason for adopting this focus is that there has been relatively little work that tackles the challenge head-on. Surveying the field, there is a large and growing body of work on pastoral and ecclesial practice in relation to dementia, which, while valuable and worthy of acknowledgment, is not particularly relevant here.[8] There is a smaller but enormously important body of work on the experience of dementia for Christians living with it, along with their theological reflections on the experience.[9] But the doctrinal implications of dementia are much less well covered, with the majority of distinctly theological contributions taking the form of chapters in edited or co-authored volumes or individual journal articles exploring themes such as relationality,[10] self-emptying,[11] God's faithfulness,[12] and Christ's solidarity.[13] Book-length treatments of the theology of dementia are even rarer, with only three making a substantial contribution to the field.[14]

This seems a pity, and I will make the argument that the experience of dementia forces us to theologize creatively and boldly because it has several

---

7. Cook, "Lived Experience," 84.

8. See, e.g., Baxley and Goldsmith, "In a Strange Land"; Van De Creek, *Spiritual Care*; Atwell et al., *God in Fragments*; Collicutt, *Thinking of You*.

9. E.g., Bryden, *Who Will I Be When I Die?*; Bryden, "Spiritual Journey"; Bute and Morse, *Dementia from the Inside*; Davis and Davis, *My Journey*; Williams, *What Happens to Faith*.

10. Williams, "Knowing God in Dementia."

11. Cook, "Lived Experience."

12. Hudson, "God's Faithfulness."

13. Kevern, "Sharing the Mind of Christ."

14. Keck, *Forgetting*; Mast, *Second Forgetting*; Swinton, *Dementia*.

distinctive features. In the first place, intellectual disabilities present themselves to us as more theologically challenging than physical ones because they seem to strike at our capacity for faith: if one cannot hear and understand the gospel, how may one be saved? Secondly, as an acquired and progressive family of conditions, dementia differs from cognitive impairment that is part of the constitution of the individual from birth: we have to deal with the change in condition and with the consequent uncertainty about what has happened to the person we used to know. We can deal with the theological questions surrounding people born with a cognitive impairment who therefore may not develop a "typical" set of adult intellectual attributes by reference (whether this is justified or not) to the theological status of babies or small children; but this cannot apply in the same way to adults who have lived full, committed, faith-filled lives and in whom this faith history seems to be being erased. Finally, therefore, we have to deal with the fact of dementia as an *event*, one that on the face of it lacks all theological meaning or salience, since it is the loss of meaning itself. For all these reasons, dementia can lay claim to be the preeminent "theological disease."[15]

So this book is ultimately not about dementia but about theology—or at least about theology seen through the lens of dementia. Like much good theology (and some bad theology too) it has its roots in a human story, or a succession of stories, about my mother's dementia:[16] starting from personal experience it works outward and upward, from phenomenology to theology.[17]

---

15. Keck, *Forgetting*, 17.

16. Throughout the book I will refer to mum, my mother, and Daphne at different points, depending on whether I am thinking about her in relationship to me or seeking to emphasize her independent status.

17. I.e., reflecting on the shape of our experience of dementia as the starting-point for our theology. "Unlike approaches in the social sciences, phenomenology is not primarily concerned with empirical experience—how this or that person might experience a specific event at a particular moment—but rather with the broader structures of experience in order to ascertain what sort or kind of experience it is, its various modes of manifestation, and how it reveals something about the human condition." Gschwandtner, "Mystery Manifested," 315.

Introduction

> Mum first began to complain of symptoms in the mid 1990s, when she would have been in her mid sixties. With hindsight, they were the classic indicators of possible Alzheimer's—forgetfulness, repetitiveness, losing items—but we were slow to recognize them. Mum had always been prone to forgetting where she left things, and perhaps the menopause had made things worse. Mum and dad were living through changes, as he retired and they contemplated moving, so a little chaos was to be expected. And at the time, very few people were talking about dementia in younger people: clinically, it was still often referred to as "senile dementia," and colloquially, people still talked about things that made them angry as "driving me demented." In addition, relatives have a way of denying what's going on until the symptoms become unmistakable, and as a family we were no exception.
>
> Mum and dad were living in a different part of the country, so I saw them relatively rarely and did not notice how things were developing. But the presence of some condition that was affecting mum's mind became undeniable around Christmas 1998, when mum and dad were staying with my brother's family. She broke her ankle, found herself under the influence of anesthesia in an unfamiliar environment in hospital, and could not orient herself.

Touching God does not claim to be a comprehensive account of theology from the perspective of dementia, or to adopt a systematic approach to the topic. It is more in the mode of a theological journey, in which I follow a train of thought and pick up along the way whatever theological tools and resources seem to shed light on the next steps. At different points along the way, different interlocutors and ideas will come to the fore, then drop away for a while before, perhaps, reappearing at a later stage. I have treated few of them with the detailed attention and engagement that they deserve (although I hope I have misrepresented none), and deployed them only for as long as they were useful to advance the thinking process. The result is a very personal theological account and absolutely not the last word on the subject: but it may at least be a conversation starter, an initial scouting expedition through the territory, and perhaps even a provocation to encourage others to attempt to tread their own way through.

> The next point I remember along the way was on our wedding day in 1999, when mum was bright, engaged and seemingly well on top of the situation. I said as much to my dad when we were leaving, and he agreed; but told me that by the end of the day she would not remember any of the events. As mum's symptoms developed, they became more visible in social contexts. We have a set of photographs from a day out around 2000 in which she is smiling brightly at the camera, but there is something unfocused in her gaze: she is not sure where she is, or who is around her.
>
> But there is another picture from one Christmas about the same time, where mum is laughing and looking at me. She clearly loves me and loves being with me, although at that time she would not have been able to name me as her son without prompting. And there were sudden moments of clarity, such as the time when she asked me what I was working on (something technical and self-indulgent on the possibility of Christian polytheism) and was suddenly engaged, understanding, and critically acute in her response. It was the moment I recognized her as my first and best theological mentor.

The question of what dementia might *mean* theologically has been nagging at me for about the last twenty years, and I think that it boils down to three convictions that need to be held together when we think about dementia.

The first is that *dementia doesn't change anything fundamental about the believer*. Of course, all sorts of attributes change and many of the practices and beliefs we associate with being a believer become impossible or irrelevant; but the status of the person before God does not change. The encounter with dementia does not impair or prevent somebody's Christian faith, so we need to find ways of understanding that faith that are hospitable to our understanding of dementia.

INTRODUCTION

> Nevertheless, in that period, as my brother put it, "the islands of memory" were becoming separated from each other in my mother's mind: she was losing the capacity to link them together into a coherent narrative, to navigate her way around spaces, to complete some basic tasks without help. In the same way she was losing her cognitive capacity, self-agency, and social self. My dad was taking increasing responsibility for their domestic life, organizing life around her, prompting her memory and providing care where needed. Mum remained recognizably herself: bright, funny, loving, and clearly devoted to her faith. Only those who knew her well would have noticed that her responses often hid the fact that she didn't necessarily know what was going on and was increasingly reliant on a diminishing set of stock phrases.

Secondly, I contend that dementia *doesn't change anything about God*. This seems too obvious to be worth mentioning, but I intend to show that if we take dementia with full theological seriousness, we are going to have to revise some of our thinking about what sort of a God allows, uses, and perhaps even values the event of dementia in the life of a believing person. Specifically, if we believe Jesus's promise that "I am with you always, to the very end of the age,"[18] we must ask what that means in practice, if we experience dementia as a sort of abandonment in the "Bad Home."

> Mum's faith remained firm even as her grasp of its content and forms slipped away. There was a period in which, whenever we met, she would insist that we prayed. We would put our hands together and bow our heads, and she would adopt a "prayerful" voice as she led us in devotions that did not "make sense" in sentences or even complete words. But they made sense to her, it seems.
>
> As her dementia progressed further, mum became less able to be left alone for any period of time, less able to perform the basic tasks of dressing and going to the toilet unaided and, increasingly, resistant to dad's help with those intimate tasks as she became less able to recognize him. He in turn became isolated, exhausted, and sad, mourning the woman whose love he seemed to have lost and the future he had hoped they still had together.

---

18. Matt 28:20.

Faith in the constancy of God leads to the third commitment, which is that *a life lived with dementia is one full of theological significance that tells us something important.* This is more controversial: while there is an abundance of books addressing the question of how Christians may cope with dementia or asserting that God loves us regardless, it is a rather different thing to state its positive significance. The very term itself—*dementia*, loss of *mens* (mind)—is expressive of a negation, and it is not immediately obvious how a negation can have positive theological significance. But if the relationship with God is unimpaired in the journey of dementia despite the loss of so many of its apparent features, dementia is telling us something important about how that relationship is constructed, maintained, and perhaps even consummated.

> My last memory of mum is from a week or so before she died, and I still have the photograph. She is in a wheelchair, having now lost the ability to walk, to speak, or to engage in any intentional activity. She is staring blankly, with no apparent interaction with her environment. And yet on her last day, my dad found she had somehow got onto her knees beside her bed. He always believed that, as she heard God's call, she prepared herself for death. Mum died on the third of April 2004, at the age of seventy-five.

These three commitments are expanded upon and explored through the chapters of this book. But as well as being an exploration of what dementia means for our understanding of God (and vice versa), this book is also the working out of a method (or perhaps a cautionary tale). It illustrates what can happen when somebody finds a nagging question, a loose thread, and won't stop pulling at it regardless of where it leads theologically. What has resulted in this case is not systematic, and does not attempt to be comprehensive. Like a neuron embedded in a healthy brain, it branches in a number of different directions and makes connections that can appear almost random. The elements of a constructive theology of dementia can be connected in many different ways, the possible routes linking them are almost infinite, and in this book I refer in passing to a few roads not traveled. It is my hope that others will pick up where it leaves off, to challenge, refute, or develop some more ideas on how we make sense theologically of the questions posed.

INTRODUCTION

Summary of chapters

The title of this book (*Touching God*) reflects a growing conviction in me that, if we want to talk about the relationship between somebody who lives with dementia and their God, the metaphor of *touch* provides a more fertile point of departure than those of speaking and listening, or action and response, or seeing and knowing. Touch is the first of our senses to provide a point of communication in the newborn, and the process of touching and being touched is the basis for our earliest contact with the world, as well as the source of our profoundest attachments. For people living with advanced dementia, it is usually also the last sense to be lost, even if there is no human contact, as there is the sensation of air in our lungs, the movements of our organs, and the pressure of gravity on our bodies. Furthermore, it is a sensory experience from which we cannot distance ourselves, and from which we cannot be separated. It seems, then, that the phenomenon of bodily touch is the most appropriate way to explore the interface between us and God: particularly because, as I go on to argue, the Incarnate Christ meets us "body to body." It is a small step from that realization to the decision to think about the relationship between us and God in the midst of dementia in terms of three "bodies" of Christ, ways in which Christ is present to us physically, ecclesially, and sacramentally, in anticipation of the eschaton in which we will ourselves be resurrected. This overarching theme of the "three bodies" of Christ (which has ancient origins and was explored in great detail by Henri de Lubac)[19] emerged into prominence for me late in the writing process and helps to give shape and direction to the whole.

The perspective I am taking is as a practicing Catholic, and for some of the subject matter (such as the treatment of the Eucharist) I have taken an unapologetically Catholic position. However, the chapters and therefore their treatment of their topics vary in style and approach, partly because they have their origins in different times and challenges, and partly because different topics require different tools. For the same reasons, they draw on and engage in depth with different authors or sources of inspiration. The overall effect, I hope, is of a series of panels in a painted screen: each of them stands alone and can be read without much reference to the others, but together they give an overview of the landscape that is greater than the sum of its parts.

---

19. De Lubac, *Corpus Mysticum*.

The first chapter begins by unpacking why the thought of dementia has such a tight grip on our collective psyche: why it seems uniquely able to inspire in us a deep dread. I trace the roots of that dread to our understanding of what makes a human being, and argue that to be delivered from it requires an understanding of human beings "before God": a theological anthropology. This leads into a discussion of each of us as being created in the image of God, and an exploration of what that might mean in the face of dementia. It concludes that we cannot understand how a person with dementia can be thought of as in the image of God without a clear understanding of how God is involved with all of our life, from beginning to end.

Chapter 2 therefore begins with the question of what we need to say about God in order to say something theologically meaningful about the personhood of somebody living with dementia. In it I develop the thought that any God who is meaningful for a person living with dementia is, in turn, one for whom a life lived with dementia is meaningful. In other words, God is involved in the history of that person: the struggles, changes, challenges, and triumphs in the life of a person with dementia are part of their relationship with God. This leads us to a consideration of Christology, of Christ as both God-in-history and our human exemplar as we seek to grow into the divine likeness. The conclusion of the chapter is that in order to talk of the experience of dementia as theologically meaningful, we must bring it into an encounter with Christ-in-our-history. This entails the notion of Christ as present to us in three "bodies": as a historical fleshly body, as the ecclesial body, and as the sacrament that is the presence of his resurrected body.

Chapter 3 develops this theme by exploring how, in the passion narrative of Jesus Christ, we may identify the work of a God who, in turn, identifies with our frailty. The tone of this chapter is more meditative as it retells the narrative of Christ's sufferings as one in which he shares in our sufferings even to the point of "losing his mind" in acute delirium. The true identity of Christ is manifested at the point in which he loses his "identity" to external eyes: he is "The Incarnate, Deconstructed" who provides an answer to what Keck terms the "Deconstruction Incarnate"[20] encountered in the experience of dementia. The breaking-down of Christ's personhood in the passion also, metaphorically, creates the soil in which the Church[21] is to

---

20. Keck, *Forgetting*, 21.

21. Throughout this chapter and elsewhere in the book, I capitalize the word *Church* when I am referring to the theological concept of the completed body of Christ, and use

Introduction

grow: those who witness the process, take his fleshly body from the cross, are the last to touch his flesh, and become the nucleus of his ecclesial body.

Chapter 4 picks up these thoughts in a more practical mode, enquiring about the place of people with dementia within the Church and its implications. It works with the disjunction between the church as social institution and the Church as the mystical body of Christ, and explores how the ecclesial body of Christ can only be manifest when the institutional church steps outside its own boundaries to recognize its dependence on marginalized people such as those living with dementia. These ideas are developed in critical conversation with a seventh-century biography of a sixth-century saint, Symeon of Emesa.

Chapter 5 continues this problem-based approach by analyzing a well-known case study, the story of the "Lost Mariner," in the light of contemporary sacramental theology. The chapter draws upon the work of some recent philosophers in the Continental phenomenological tradition to consider how we, in our bodiliness, encounter God in the sacramental body of Christ; and how this encounter may give us a deeper understanding of God's presence to us in a life lived with dementia. Some fertile ideas emerge in this discussion, in particular Marion's understanding of Christ's self-emptying in the eucharistic elements, and how it calls forth from us a self-emptying in response. The question arises of whether the experience of dementia may itself be understood as an emptying of this sort and, if so, how the journey to union with God may be understood to continue in and through dementia.

Chapters 6 and 7 develop the theme of a journey to God through dementia, and how it may be understood. Chapter 6 focuses on the middle stages of dementia, when abstract thinking is becoming more difficult, care needs are increasing, and language is progressively being lost. Drawing on the testimonies of people living with dementia, it explores what may be opening up as, on the face of it, their world is closing down, and identifies two possible areas of growth. The first is that, as cognitive capacities decline, some people with dementia report a new and unmediated emotional intimacy with God, an encounter at an organic level. The second is that the progressive loss of language does not seem to equate to a progressive loss of religious meanings, but the sudden arrival of new and uncontrolled ones in an explosion of metaphor. Together, these findings suggest that God

---

the lowercase *church* when I am discussing social and historical groups of Christians and their institutions.

continues to draw close, and the person continues to respond, but in new and more naked ways.

Chapter 7 is, on the face of it, bleaker: it attempts to understand what might be going on during late-stage dementia, when communication is all but impossible and there may be no discernible awareness of or response to surroundings. In an attempt to understand what "touching God" might mean in the face of what has been called "the blank Alzheimer's stare," we turn back to the fleshly body of Christ, and specifically the theology of Christ's incarnation as understood by some of the great theologians of the Church. The picture that emerges is of Christ as intimately bound to us at every level, including (and perhaps especially) our physical flesh.

Having moved full circle back to a (revised and broadened) understanding of the fleshly body of Christ as intimately associated with our own flesh, chapter 8 considers our future destiny as resurrected bodies in communion with Christ's body, in order to review the journey of life with dementia against an eschatological horizon. The central themes developed in this chapter are that resurrection must entail complete dependence on our communion with Christ and our social networks "in Christ" and that therefore the progress from time to eternity needs to be understood as a move from mundane completeness to radical incompleteness, not vice versa. There are implications for how we are to understand the theological significance of living with dementia: the process of "dying again, and again, and again" is at the same time an anticipation of and preparation for an eternity of communion in God.

This brings us to the concluding chapter, and a review of where the journey has taken us. I argue here that the three commitments with which the book began are resolved in a vision of Christ who is with us "body to body" in all times and in all ways, and in whom we in turn are embraced at the end of time and space. Within that vision, some recurrent themes are teased out and looked at again: the way in which Christ is manifest at the point of a loss of his "identity"; the answering call to incompleteness and *kenosis* in our growth into the divine likeness; and the assurance that, in discovering the incompleteness heralded and symbolized by the journey into dementia, we can have hope in perfect communion with God.

This was not the book I intended to write, and I offer it with some trepidation. Although I had a fairly clear idea that it would be exploring the meaning of dementia in the light of the incarnation, most of the key themes and lines of thought emerged organically in the process. Some of them still

Introduction

feel unfamiliar to me, poorly integrated with the main tenets of Christian dogma, and in need of much more work. At best, they may provide a seam of ideas that can be applied to related fields where disability or impairment pose theological questions; at worst, they may prove misleading and create unhelpful confusion.

In addition, I am keenly aware of the limitations of this book, relying as it does mostly on my own experiences and written resources. Many people who live with dementia, and many others who have experience of accompanying them on the journey, will not recognize their experience in the account I have given here. I can justly be accused of underplaying the distress, the confusion, the sheer exhaustion and despair that frequently dominate the experience both of the person themselves and those close to them, and taking a position that is too detached and cerebral. My only defense here is that there are already plenty of books detailing the turmoil that accompanies dementia, but not very many that try to make sense of it "after the dust has settled." It is far from complete, but I hope it harms nobody, and may even be useful for some.

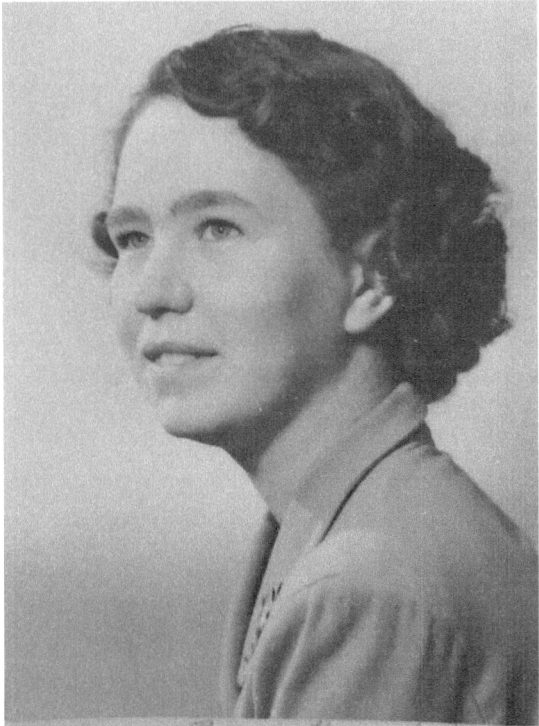

Daphne Kevern, 1928–2004

1

Why are we so afraid of dementia?

> Mum first died on the 12th of May 2019
>   when she couldn't work out how to prepare her legendary roast anymore.
> The style icon of the Covington estate,
>   Mum died as a fashionista the day she couldn't get dressed into her colorful outfits . . . .
> She died as the Queen of Christmas
>   when she refused to have dinner with the family.
> She died again when she asked me,
>   her son, what my name was.
> She died as Dad's Rock,
>   after fifty-two years of marriage,
>   the day she looked straight through him.
> On 10th March 2024,
>   Mum died a final time,
>   surrounded by her family.
>
> *With dementia, you don't just die once, you die again, and again, and again.*[1]

WHEN IN MARCH 2024 the Alzheimer's Society (the UK's largest and most influential dementia charity) released this advert on television, radio, and social media, it was to a flurry of debate and bafflement. Responses (still recorded and recoverable on the Alzheimer's Society Facebook page and

---

1. Alzheimer's Society, "Long Goodbye." I am indebted to Joanna Collicutt for drawing my attention to the advert and debate around it.

in response to the YouTube postings) were bewilderingly diverse, but almost uniformly impassioned.² For some, this was a crass and insensitive representation of dementia that frightened those recently diagnosed or caring for somebody living with the condition; that undid years of messaging about the possibility and necessity of "living well" with dementia; and that neglected the many ways in which (in their experience) loved ones continued to "be themselves" despite the losses and deficits. For others, the advert was no more than an honest, unflinching look at the brutal reality of loving somebody disappearing before their eyes, dissolving under the onslaught of a condition David Keck memorably called, "deconstruction incarnate."³ In the opinion of the Society's CEO, who in the light of the criticism was moved to respond, the film was an opportunity to tell the stories of people whose lives had been affected by dementia, "raising awareness of the devastating reality of dementia for so many families." It was a shout for attention, because "Every time we shy away from talking about it, we give policy makers and decision makers cover to ignore dementia and take action on something else. It's just not good enough, dementia isn't the priority it should be, and we can't put up with it anymore."⁴

What comes through clearly in the advert and all these reactions to it is the emotional intensity that accompanies the subject, the sense that the very dignity of human beings is at stake in the way we talk of, think about, and respond to it. Dementia is consistently emerging as the most feared disease of all among older people in the UK, USA, and Australia,⁵ and its capacity to inspire a sort of existential dread (as Michael Aylwin puts it, "It comes for your very soul")⁶ almost certainly explains the imaginative power that it exerts over Western societies. For the same reason, it needs to be treated seriously as a topic for theological reflection: as we dig down to the sources of our collective dread, we will gain insight into what are for us the "matters of ultimate concern,"⁷ how they are structured and how (if at all) they align with the Christian theological tradition.

---

2. See "The Long Goodbye" on YouTube for a selection of responses.
3. Keck, *Forgetting*, 21.
4. Alzheimer's Society, "CEO Responds."
5. Watson et al., "Second Most Feared Condition"; Alzheimer's Research UK, "Dementia Attitudes"; UsAgainstAlzheimer's, "Alzheimer's Disease Crisis."
6. Aylwin, "'It Comes for Your Very Soul.'"
7. Tillich, *Systematic Theology*, 234.

In this chapter I will begin by exploring the features of this dread—what drives it, what feeds it—by reflecting on some of the key messages hidden in the short passage with which I opened the chapter. I will then point to ways in which scholars, practitioners, and people who themselves live with dementia have resisted the "deconstruction" embedded in the encounter with dementia and sought to meaningfully reconstruct personhood in the face of the condition. Finally, I will consider how a response to the theological challenge of dementia requires us to retrieve and rethink in what sense we are in the image of God and, conversely, the sort of God whose image we are. This will prepare the ground for the chapter to follow.

Delving deeper: The hypercognitive society

Mum first died on the 12th of May 2019
when she couldn't work out how . . .

If we dread dementia because it rouses our existential fear of death itself, then we need to examine what we think is dying.[8] If I fear that dementia will rob me of whatever "makes me myself," then we may want to examine our assumptions about what that is.

The classic answer is that what is dying is the "inner self," the "true identity" that thinks, feels, acts, and remembers in an inner space that needs to be maintained and protected. There are two dimensions here: we imagine that each of us has a "true self" that exists independently of everybody else in an inner space; and that we know about this "true self" because it performs mental actions in the abstract, apart from the world around us. This understanding of what makes me myself is embedded in a long tradition of Western thinking about the nature of the person, beginning perhaps with Plato, mediated to the West through Boethius's understanding of the primacy of reason,[9] and becoming popularized in Rene Descartes's famous formula, *Cogito ergo sum*, "I think, therefore I am."[10] My very being is to be found in my capacity to think, and from that develops my self-consciousness, my capacity for intentional action, and my interactions with the world around me. And although Western understandings of what makes a person have expanded out from this narrow base to include the importance of

---

8. Bryden, *Dancing*, 159.
9. Comensoli, *In God's Image*, 29.
10. Descartes, *Discourse on Method*, 53.

self-narrative (Locke), the will to power (Nietzsche), decision and choice (Kierkegaard and Sartre), they have, with very few exceptions, remained with the starting-point of an individual making intentional decisions from a self-conscious core.

The upshot of our inadequate understanding of personhood is that, without consciously intending to, we have found ourselves in a "hyper-cognitive" society,[11] in which "the image of human fulfilment is framed by cognition and productivity."[12] We understand ourselves as a bundle of shifting functions and roles held together by an isolated inner self that reflects, chooses, and molds the coherent narrative that comprises our personhood, the thread of continuity that persists over the course of our life. Dementia strikes at the heart of what we consider to be "us": our ability to think coherently, to find a truth at our center, from which we can be ourselves in whatever we do in a shifting world. If our "soul" is our cognitive self, it is no surprise that we are afraid of dementia, and that our only hope is that a new generation of drugs may restore some level of cognitive function and so "save our souls."

This is not just a misconception we nurture as individuals, but a reflection on a flaw in our society as a whole. According to Stephen Post's analysis of the problem, our fear of dementia exposes the sub-Christian values that have permeated our understanding of what it is to be a human person. It turns out that we value people in secular, rather than Christian ways, because we have become wedded to the essentially Stoic values of control, thrift, rationality, and success. Instead, he says, we have to "enlarge our sense of human worth to counter an exclusionary emphasis on rationality, efficient use of time and energy, ability to control distracting impulses, thrift, economic success, self-reliance, 'language advantage,' and the like."[13]

It needs to be pointed out at this stage that both our experience of dementia and our dread of it appear to be very strongly influenced by this cultural background. Western society is virtually unique in recognizing dementia as distinct from the normal and inevitable process of aging; in its emphasis on rationality as the seat of human personhood; and in its understanding of human beings as, primarily, distinct individuals. For good or ill, many other societies have no term in their language for dementia, construct their understanding of personhood more in terms of relationships than

11. Post, "Concept of Alzheimer Disease."
12. Post, *Moral Challenge*, 34.
13. Post, "Respectare," 233.

individual attributes, and value different competencies or contributions to society.[14] Objectively, the dread that we may feel and the sense of death that appears to haunt our experience of dementia are reflections of the society in which we find ourselves. This gives us hope: perhaps, by learning to see differently, we may see more truly.

Might we be able to confront our dread and understand it better if we look at the problem from the other end? What happens if we *start* by affirming that we love and recognize the personhood of the person in front of us, and only then start worrying about what attributes and capacities they have? What would it be like to live in a society that will value me as a person *before* it starts to specify what I need to be and to do in order to "qualify"? This is the approach taken by a family of "personalist" philosophies that "regard the person as the ultimate explanatory, epistemological, ontological, and axiological principle of all reality" prior to any assumptions about what being a person entails.[15] If we affirm this strongly enough, then the existential question of whether the person with dementia is "still there" becomes reduced to a practical one, of how we *recognize* the person whom we have already decided is there, even if they are present in a way that is unfamiliar to us. This *a priori* assertion enables talk of the rights and dignity of people with dementia without becoming enmeshed in questions of how their personhood is seen or overlooked by other people.[16]

The main problem with secular personalist approaches is that personalism lacks any grounding other than as a bare assertion. As Williams and Bengtsson point out, personalism may be derived from a prior metaphysics but cannot provide that metaphysics in itself. An assertion that all people living with dementia are fully and completely persons regardless of their impairment may be advanced, but may just as easily be withdrawn if the mood changes, because there is nothing else "at stake" that affects those not sharing in the condition. There are some interesting attempts to overcome this difficulty—notably Fuchs's phenomenological account of human beings as comprised of a sedimented history and internalized set of social relations that are inscribed in "body memory" as well as in the (impaired) conscious, reflective memory[17]—but even this, ultimately, falters when the pre-reflective level of agency and response is no longer discernible.

14. Ekoh et al., "Appraisal of Public Understanding."
15. Williams and Bengtsson, "Personalism."
16. Treanor, *Intellectual Disability*.
17. Fuchs, "Embodiment and Personal Identity in Dementia."

Personalism, then, needs a grounding in theology: we need to have a *reason* to believe that a person with profound dementia is nevertheless still with us, and it is notable that personalism was developed with input from some significant twentieth-century theologians (notably Jacques Maritain and Pope John II).[18] Theologically, human identity does not come from some metaphysical essence nor our social assumptions, but is conferred and maintained by God. We need a theology of what it is to be a person, if we are to anchor these claims in anything other than a pious yearning.

The social self

> *She died as the Queen of Christmas*
> *when she refused to have dinner with the family.*

Examining the passage with which this chapter opened, we can see that there are two senses to the statement that "Mum died" while she was still physically alive. On the surface, it seems to be about her individual subjectivity, the inner spark that makes her herself. However, on closer examination we can see that most of the references to dying are to "social death," to the ways in which social connections and other peoples' understanding of her as a person are being lost.[19]

When we talk about personhood, we tend to think of a person as an independent maker of meaning, creating their self-narrative in isolation. But there is a substantial sociological tradition that stresses the importance of social connections in this process.[20] In the phraseology of African Ubuntu philosophy, "I am because we are."[21] We may even say that the "inner self" that I think I am is not my own property but is only lent to me by the community surrounding me. All of us emerge from the womb unformed as individuals, and are "loved into shape" by those around us (and children cut off from this contact in their early years typically fail to develop as individuals). Similarly, we may say that as our capacity to maintain our sense of self falters through frailty and cognitive loss, it is others who take back responsibility for our sense of self, reminding us of our social network and our place within it. My personhood was never, purely and simply, my

---

18. Williams and Bengtsson, "Personalism."
19. Sweeting and Gilhooly, "Social Death."
20. E.g., Durkheim, *Division of Labour*.
21. Ogude, *Ubuntu and Personhood*.

own: "Identity . . . stands in a dialectical relationship with society. Identity is formed by social processes. Once crystallized, it is maintained, modified, or even reshaped by social relations."[22]

This two-way relationship between individuality and society has particular relevance when, as in the case of someone with dementia, personhood seems to be changing. More than thirty years ago, Stephen Sabat pointed out that the "I" is a complex construct, encompassing three distinct senses of self: Self 1 (personal identity, my personal point of view), Self 2 (the mental and physical attributes I have at present), and Self 3, comprising all the "selves" I am in relation to others.[23] All of us rely on the community for our sense of self, but this is particularly the case as my cognitive capacity diminishes through age, frailty, or dementia, since it will be Self 3 that will necessarily predominate, and the community's respect and memories of me that will maintain me as an individual. Responsibility for "conscious, collective authorship of the self-narrative"[24] will pass increasingly from me to those around me. It should come as no surprise, then, that within the field of dementia care a lot of attention has been paid to the way in which our social context preserves, or undermines, our personhood along with the networks and the memories, the roles and narratives that comprise such a significant part of it.

The decisive contribution here was made by the work of Tom Kitwood, who in his seminal 1997 book *Dementia Reconsidered* took issue with the narrowly clinical understanding of dementia that was largely unchallenged at that time. He argued that many of the observed deficits and symptoms of dementia were not of clinical origin but due to the "malignant social psychology" of the people who comprise the person's social network, and their often well-meaning attempts to help. As he pointed out, much of what appears at first to be "help" has the effect of disempowering or erasing the personhood of the person concerned, to their detriment. Hence, he subtitled his book *The Person Comes First*, and was largely responsible for the movement toward "person-centered care" that grew up in the following decade.[25]

As a person's dementia progresses and communication becomes more difficult, so their social networks change also, and Kitwood's work has led

---

22. Berger and Luckmann, *Social Construction of Reality*, 194.
23. Sabat, *Experience*, 17–18.
24. Radden and Fordyce, "Into the Darkness," 71–88.
25. Kitwood, *Dementia Reconsidered*.

to much more attention and energy being directed to restoring or maintaining this social dimension of the self. Welcoming social networks such as the European Meeting Centres program[26] and the Church of England's Dementia Friendly Churches initiatives[27] can support the person living with dementia both directly by providing social support and indirectly by "caring for the carers" so that the person's closest associates can continue with the "active, collective authorship of the self-narrative." When such narration seems to be impossible due to loss of coherence, memory, and language, Julie Simpson's impressive PhD work has shown how a detailed and "ethnographic" involvement with the individual, their personal history and their community, can enable a sensitive and fruitful response to their existential needs.[28] Social death is not, it appears, an inevitable consequence of the onset of dementia.

However, Kitwood's own commitment to empowering and humanizing social interaction may have left him blind to the way that imbalances of power may (deliberately or inadvertently) crush or appropriate the social self. Several writers have noted that his account of the person, taken on its own, is non-realist and strangely ungrounded. There is a danger that, when "collaborative authorship of the self-narrative" moves from the individual to the community, the person disappears in a fanciful construction.[29] They may be "re-narrated" by others: made recipients of others' projections and assumptions about what the person's "real self" is like to the extent that they are not allowed to change and develop as their dementia progresses.[30] Among those who love and are close to the person with dementia, there is typically an element of denial, a desire to maintain that nothing has changed, to cling to the person they once were. But everybody changes, and an insistence that their tastes, preferences, and choices are immutable can be its own sort of oppression. Here there is another example of what Kitwood refers to as "malignant social psychology": the mechanism by which

---

26. Meeting Centres UK, "Evidence."
27. Kevern and Primrose, "Changes in Measures," 337.
28. Simpson, "*I Still.*"
29. Thornton, "Discursive Turn," 140.
30. Chapman, Philip, and Komesaroff, "Person-Centred Problem." As my colleague Dr. Edward Tolhurst points out, this loss of the ability to change one's self-narrative is at the bottom of Sartre's phrase "Hell is other people" (*l'enfer c'est les autres*)!

our unreflective assumptions and poorly handled attempts to "help" may end up alienating and disempowering the very person we want to support.[31]

So, in response to the peculiar and painful vulnerability that accompanies the development of dementia by somebody we love, we need to come to an understanding of the human person that does not depend on a remembered construction of their "real self" but a sense of what they are here for and where they are heading, supported by what John Swinton calls a community of attentiveness.[32] This is a theological issue, resting as it does on the mystery of what we are, what we are created to be, and how we are to journey between the two. It also requires us to consider the language we use when we talk about dementia and those living with it, since it is this which will shape the narrative that we construct. This brings us to the question of language: how do we talk about persons, and how do we talk about how dementia affects them?

Talking of dementia and the person as the "living dead"

With dementia, you don't just die once, you die again, and again, and again.

The choice of language in the advert we are examining matters, because it "positions" the subject of the eulogy in a particular way that can influence their existential wellbeing. When it comes to dementia, the language itself reflects and feeds our dread. It is filled with images of warfare: of mind-robbers, attacks, and strikes by an alien invader.[33] Behuniak points to the way the metaphor of the "zombie"—as someone whose personhood has departed, leaving behind an animated body of decaying flesh that refuses to die—has been deployed in popular media discourse around dementia,[34] with a similar range of metaphors commonplace across literature, film, and news media.[35]

It is possible to interpret this curious use of dehumanizing language as expressive of our relentless search for imagery that will grab our attention and monetize it; but it also has a political and intentional aspect. Thus, in

---

31. Kitwood, *Dementia Reconsidered*.
32. Swinton, *Dementia*.
33. George, "Art of Medicine."
34. Behuniak, "Living Dead?"
35. Low and Purwaningrum, "Negative Stereotypes."

her defense of the language of "dying again, and again, and again" in the advert, the CEO of the Alzheimer's Society points to its potential to force the hand of policy makers: "Every time we shy away from talking about it, we give policy makers and decision makers cover to ignore dementia and take action on something else."[36] Similarly, Megan-Jane Johnstone has argued from her deep dive into the Australian media environment that the use of a narrative of invasion, injury, loss, and dehumanization about dementia both fuels and is driven by the debate on assisted dying.[37] Our discourse on meaning, purpose, and value is one in which existential anxiety about dementia is only one of the forces competing for our attention and seeking to shape the language world in which we move.

Much of our language has the effect of treating the person with dementia as an "other," lacking the markers of human identity and therefore an occasion for fear and distancing.[38] It is not easy to treat someone as a person with full dignity if the label "zombie" has been attached to them. It is almost impossible to contribute to the "conscious, collective authorship of the self-narrative" if the narrative is of invasion or "hollowing out" of the person. In general, then, it seems very likely that the language that we develop to express our fears and to cope with the progress of dementia in ourselves and others actually "locks us in" to that way of thinking, ultimately amplifying our fears while closing off other ways of thinking that may open up new hope. "Part of our moral challenge in adapting to ageing populations is about semantic choice. . . . Specifically, our societal perspective might be less distressing if individuals and their families could see dementia not just as a 'loss of self,' but as a change in self not so unlike many others a person undergoes in other life stages."[39]

For this reason, at the level of the language and rhetoric around dementia, many carers and support workers have made conscious efforts to shift the language from the impersonal to the personal, and from the passive to the active.[40] The language used has evolved over the last forty years from references to, collectively, "the demented" (who appear to have no

---

36. Alzheimer's Society, "CEO Responds."
37. Johnstone, "Metaphors"; Johnstone, *Alzheimer's Disease*.
38. Naue and Kroll, "'Demented Other'"; Sabat et al., "'Demented Other' or Simply 'a Person'?"
39. George, "Art of Medicine," 587.
40. Mason et al., "Language."

personhood at all)[41] to "demented people" (who have personhood, but are defined primarily by their condition)[42] to "people living with dementia" (who are not only persons, but active agents who are not circumscribed by their dementia),[43] and even "people living well with dementia" (to stress that it is not merely a "death sentence" but opens up a new phase of life).[44] As well as consciously counteracting the depersonalized, non-agentic "zombie" language prevalent in popular discourse, this shift in terminology restores the person, their agency, and their needs to the front and center of the conversation and so lays the groundwork for sustained attention to their existential needs.

Confronting our dread begins with the language that is used, both in reference and in conversation: the discourse must change, and we must find a meaning or language for dementia that is other than a "defectology."[45] But the brute fact is that, from any earthly perspective, the progression of dementia presents itself as a series of deficits and losses that cannot be reversed, and that end in death. Any response must reach into the heart of loss and death itself to find meaning and purpose, acknowledging rather than denying them: anything else is just a lie, the construction of a flimsy screen to hide the too-frightening reality of our condition. Dementia brings us up hard against the meaning of loss and death, and this makes our search for language a theological project from top to bottom.

On *not* dying "again, and again, and again"

This analysis of the advert has laid bare some of the dimensions of the experience of dementia represented by "dying again, and again, and again" and so helps to point us to some of the essential theological challenges. However, our analysis would be incomplete if we did not briefly acknowledge the work of some creative and courageous people who have lived with the condition and who reject the sentence of dementia as an endless series of dyings. Three well-known examples may help to make this point.

41. Baumgarten, "Health of Persons."
42. Naue and Kroll, "'Demented Other.'"
43. Mason et al., "Language."
44. Kim and Shin, "'Living Well' Concept."
45. The term is used by Swinton to indicate how people living with dementia and others are defined by their assumed failure to conform to the criteria of "normality." See Swinton, *Dementia*, 41–42.

First, there is Christine Bryden, who I referred to earlier in this chapter. She was a senior scientist working with the Australian government when she started to display the first symptoms of dementia; now, some twenty-five years on, she continues to write and speak on the subject. By virtue of this unusual trajectory, she brings to her account of the experience her advanced communicative ability and her extended reflection on the meaning of what is happening to her:

> Dementia is often thought of as death by small steps, but we must ask ourselves what is really dying. Hasn't the person with dementia reached that place of "now," of existing actively in the present? . . . I believe that people with dementia are making an important journey from cognition, through emotion, into spirit. I've begun to realize what really remains throughout this journey is what is really important, and what disappears is what is not important. I think that if society could appreciate this, then people with dementia would be respected and treasured.[46]

If for Bryden the way to existential wellbeing was via a letting-go and active living in the present, for Wendy Mitchell the response was almost the opposite. She used her considerable organizational and planning skills (honed as a non-clinical manager in the NHS) to compensate for the growing deficits and to maintain control over her life for more than ten years, chronicling her progress in three books (two of which so far have been best sellers). Her control extended to her choice of death, by voluntarily ceasing to eat or drink at what she considered the right time. In her final blog she wrote,

> Dementia is a cruel disease that plays tricks on your very existence. I've always been a glass half full person, trying to turn the negatives of life around and creating positives, because that's how I cope. Well I suppose dementia was the ultimate challenge. . . . Yes, dementia is a bummer, but oh what a life I've had playing games with this adversary of mine to try and stay one step ahead. . . . I didn't want dementia to take me into the later stages; that stage where I'm reliant on others for my daily needs; others deciding for me . . . . The Wendy that was didn't want to be the Wendy dementia will dictate for me.[47]

---

46. Bryden, *Dancing*, 159.
47. Mitchell, "My Final Hug."

Finally, Jennifer Bute treats her dementia not as a problem to be solved but "an unexpected gift, a wonderful opportunity and great privilege."[48] She sees it as an opportunity to contribute something distinctive and valuable to others by combining her medical knowledge as a GP with her insights as a person living with dementia within the framework of her encompassing faith. She is comfortable with the concept that the God in whom she believes ordained for her to have dementia, and she has devoted her energies to speaking, generating resources, running groups, and writing a book in order to help different communities of people to understand how to respond to people with a lived experience of dementia.[49]

In each of these cases, the person who has dementia has resisted the narrative of incremental death that structures the Alzheimer's Society advert, along with its looming threats of social death, loss of agency, and "zombification." While each is explicitly aware of their approaching physical death, they find meaning within that horizon in distinct ways, creatively reframing their experience and expanding their social networks even as some capacities are being lost. Christine Bryden finds in the incremental losses of dementia a process of simplification, enabling her to focus on what really matters in life without distraction. Wendy Mitchell exults in the excitement of the games she has had with her "adversary," rising to the challenge as a sportswoman would. Jennifer Bute finds in it a "glorious opportunity" to expand into a new dimension of discipleship. All of them subvert the grueling narrative of death; all are, in different ways, theological or a/theological responses; but all of them are irreducibly personal and particular.

As in the three examples given here, we need to develop a broader perspective on what it means, theologically, to be a person and a disciple living with dementia. The focus of the remainder of this chapter is therefore on the under-researched topic of the theological understanding of humanity that we need to ground our understanding of dementia;[50] and in the next, on the understanding of God that we need in order to make good on our claim that dementia has theological meaning and significance.

---

48. Bute, "Hello, My Name Is Jennifer Bute."
49. Bute and Morse, *Dementia from the Inside*.
50. Sloane, "Dissolving Self?"

WHY ARE WE SO AFRAID OF DEMENTIA?

Living with dementia in the image of God

For Christian theology, there is a potential grounding for a robust account of personhood in the doctrine of our creation and redemption by God. At the heart of this is the concept of the *imago Dei*, that we are created "in the image of God" so that the dignity due to God is at one remove extended also to human beings as such; and that, in Christ, we see a perfect image of what it is for us to live out that image unhindered by the effects of humanity's fall from grace.[51] Understood from this perspective, human beings do not have to *be* or *do* anything in order to qualify as the crown of God's creation: it is ours by right, by divine decree, as in the divine image. It is, we would want to say, also the birthright of absolutely everybody, including anybody living with dementia, irrespective of the types and degrees of impairment they are encountering as they journey toward communion with God.[52]

Stated like this, the doctrine of the *imago Dei* seems straightforward and of obvious use in defending the personhood of people with dementia. However, when we try to "cash out" this insight in terms of its practical range and implications, the difficulties start to multiply and force us to think more carefully. In the first place, the question immediately arises of what, in the life and experience of human beings, constitutes the image of God?[53] In the history of Jewish and Christian interpretation, three broad approaches can be discerned:

1. Substantive approaches that identify a human attribute as distinctively resembling one of God's, such as rationality, moral sense, free will, awareness of transcendence. Clearly, as soon as we try to locate the image in a particular property of the individual, we are bound to end up excluding people who don't fit our specification. The only way we could "stretch" a definition like this to include all the people we want to treat as full human beings (including the most profoundly disabled) would be to claim that sometimes the specified property is hidden: either because the person in question cannot express themselves

---

51. The key biblical passages here are Gen 1:26–27 and Col 1:15–20.

52. Comensoli, *In God's Image*, 210: "For in the end, if the profoundly impaired both are, and are meant to be, like Christ, in the same way as all other beings, then this must be reflected in how their humanity is measured."

53. This brief summary is drawn largely from Simango, "Imago Dei." A similar typology of three approaches is used by McFarland, in his detailed and systematic exposition of the topic. See *Divine Image*, 2.

sufficiently fully, or because our full glory will only be revealed at the general resurrection. In either case, we are finding space for people living with dementia in our theological framework only by putting the fact of their dementia to one side, treating them as somehow unimpaired "underneath" or "in the future." Their experience as people with dementia is stripped of its theological significance. Alternatively, we may say that the attributes that we share with God are at present obscured and marred by the effects of the fall, and will only be revealed when we are resurrected: but this just puts off the problem.[54]

Because of difficulties such as these, some disability theologians (notably Reinders) reject the appeal to *imago Dei* altogether as unhelpfully and necessarily excluding: he can conceive of it only as setting up a list of normative criteria that people with disabilities can't meet.[55] However, as I will go on to argue in chapter 8, the substantive approach still has some lessons for us. If we understand our "true nature" to be one of radical dependence on and vulnerability before God, after the example of Jesus Christ, then we may understand some people with dementia as revealing it faithfully in an exemplary way.

2. Relational approaches that identify the *imago Dei* in the human capacity to be in relationship with God and other persons. Some care needs to be taken to ensure that this capacity is not understood to be just another attribute that a person living with dementia may not possess;[56] but if instead we affirm that relationships are a given, it shifts the emphasis away from the capacities of individuals. In this study, I have started from the theological assumption that a person who has dementia continues to have a relationship with God; so if this is the basis for the claim that we are in the divine image, there should be no impediment. The question of the capacity for relationship with others is more subtle, because by definition it takes at least two to form that relationship: Could it then be concluded that a person with dementia is only in the image of God insofar as they are recognized as such by the people around them?

---

54. See the discussion in chapter 8.

55. Reinders, *Receiving*. See also Reynolds, *Vulnerable Communion*, 177.

56. So, perhaps, in Reynolds's account: "I suggest that to be created in the image of God means to be created for contributing to the world, open toward the call to love others." Reynolds, *Vulnerable Communion*, 176–77.

Worrying as this thought may be, it largely misses the point, which is that in a relational view of the *imago Dei* we can *only* be in the divine image when we are in relationship with each other. Human *individuals* are not in the image of God: human *communities* are, and this approach points us directly to our understanding of the Church. It suggests that the Church can only be understood as Christ's body, as the perfect image of God, insofar as it includes people living with a wide range of disabilities and deficits, including dementia, in meaningful relationships within it. A natural development of this approach would be to consider the redeemed relationships constituting the Church as the site in which the *imago Dei* is recognized, affirmed and made manifest.[57] This notion, that the Church only *is* the Church to the extent to which it welcomes its least "typical" members, will be explored in more detail in chapter 4.

3. Functional approaches that equate the *imago Dei* with a role, as God's representatives on earth (in the sense that a legate bearing the emperor's seal carried the emperor's authority). This is originatively the case in Adam, then preeminently the case in Jesus Christ, who is the new and undistorted Adam. Conformity between Christ's life and our life is therefore the basis of the *imago Dei*. Again, there is potential for this to be applied to a person living with dementia, although some care needs to be taken when defining what the role of a person as *imago Dei* actually is so as to avoid the excluding dynamics of the substantive approach. It would be too easy to come up with a checklist of behaviors (such as meekness and piety) that are considered "Christlike," specifying how one is to live in order to realize the *imago Dei*, and of course this would exclude people with dementia and others who may not be able to exemplify these behaviors in the accepted way.

There is however another way of understanding the fulfillment of a role: not as a set of behaviors at a particular time but as a sustained commitment, a narrative of faithfulness stretched over time that takes different forms and expressions as circumstances and capacities dictate. This is the framework that undergirds chapters 5, 6, and 7 below: that faithfulness, and so personhood in the image of God, takes different and distinct expressions as the passage of time and cognitive capacities dictate.

---

57. So Reynolds, *Vulnerable Communion*, 180–82.

There has been no systematic exploration of the implications of the concept of *imago Dei* in relation specifically to dementia, but a significant step in this direction is made by Peter Comensoli, who develops the doctrine and implications of *imago Dei* to provide an understanding of the theological status of people living with profound cognitive impairments generally. He defines the *imago Dei* as each person's call to live faithfully and fully the particular life they have been given in history, rather than conforming to a universal standard of behavior and performance: "it is the lives that human beings live, precisely in the condition in which they live it, that is significant for recognizing persons."[58]

Comensoli's approach and its development provides much of the inspiration for the remainder of this chapter. His decisive move, as we have noted, is to assert that as a result of our status in the image of God, we are persons simply because we each have a specific and God-given life to be lived, along with all the impairments we have been given as part of it. He makes some fine distinctions with care:

> They [people with profound cognitive impairments] are recognizably persons precisely because of the lives they are living in virtue of the impaired condition of their lives. The condition of their lives is not the reason they are recognizably persons, yet it is only in the condition of their lives that they can be recognizably the persons that they are.[59]

This delivers him from the charge that he is merely "stretching" the definition of the image of God to include those who would otherwise be outside it: not everybody has the same attributes, but everybody has exactly one life, so by shifting categories he has leveled the distinctions that were causing the problem.[60] He is therefore freed to reconstruct our understanding of *imago Dei*. On his account, what makes a person themselves is the fact that they are living their one life; what makes this life theologically meaningful is the fact that it is given to them by God; and it follows that the concrete historical details of that life share equally in its theological meaningfulness. Our meaning is derived from our discipleship; discipleship is a function of the life accepted in faith, this life as given by God.

This approach provides a theological grounding for the assertions that we have sought to make through the course of this chapter. It provides an

---

58. Comensoli, *In God's Image*, 2.
59. Comensoli, *In God's Image*, 3–4.
60. Comensoli, *In God's Image*, 9, 12.

alternative basis for the assertion of personhood to the "tick list" of cognitive and functional capacities that, as we have noted, are destined to be lost in the progress of dementia; one that provides the basis for a truly personalist assertion of individual worth. In addition, it provides the foundation for an understanding of social interactions that move beyond "malignant social psychology" to an affirmation of the self-narrative of the person living with dementia, insofar as that self-narrative is one of a journey toward union with God.

However, there are significant ways in which the experience of dementia raises questions that are distinct from those attending, for example, congenital cognitive impairment. From its earliest times, the Church has reflected on the status of people cognitively impaired from birth and concluded that God's grace extends to them as it does to newborn babies. But this line of thought cannot be applied in the same way to people with dementia, who may have lived long lives as mature, cognitively competent, religiously committed Christian disciples before the onset of the condition. For these subjects, the stages of life lived with dementia cannot cease to have the theological meaning and significance of the other stages, or be a retreat into childhood: as the person moves into a new stage of their Christian journey, a stage marked by the onset of dementia, so it will entail a new understanding of the God who accompanies them, and who alone gives the journey its theological meaning. As well as a theology of the person with dementia, we need a theology of the God who is present to them and of dementia itself in order to provide a new language for thinking and talking about a period of life lived with dementia, one that treats it as of equal value and potential to all other stages of life. This is a reframing, then, of our understanding of a life lived with dementia as one that is *not* "dying again, and again, and again" and that may provide us with a less dread-filled response.

In this chapter, I have argued that there are good reasons to fear dementia as a progressive and usually terminal condition that can bring with it limitation and suffering on the way to death; but that our fear is magnified by an existential dread that we will cease to be human persons by degrees along the way. To address this dread, we need to confront the assumptions about personhood that we have uncritically acquired, and find alternative ways of treating people living with dementia as fully human that do not rest on the capacities that they are losing. I went on to make the case that these alternative strategies cannot be warranted or defended without making larger claims about how human personhood may persist and even grow in the face of dementia that are in effect theological positions. I then briefly expanded on the potential of the theology of *imago Dei* to ground the claims we want to make about a person living with dementia, and pointed out the main implication: that to be living with dementia is still to be living a life freighted with theological meaning and challenge, one that is the site of redemption and of growth toward union with God.

At the end of this chapter, we have sketched out one half of a diptych. We have developed an initial understanding of persons grounded in their status as in the image of God; it now remains to us to develop a sense of the God in whose image we are in. Who is the God who bends toward us and accompanies us on the journey toward union that constitutes our claim to personhood in the image of God? This will be the main focus of the discussion to follow.

2

What sort of a God is to be found in dementia?

> He gave, and still gives me, spiritual guidance. People might say "it's a delusion, it's religious mania, it's a crutch." All I can say is this: it's my faith, my belief, that it's me that can cloud Him out. He is always faithful to me, always there when I need to say sorry. His love is constant.
>
> Without Him I am adrift, adrift in a world of darkness and fear. He allows me to be angry, to rage against Him, to question why, why, why? . . . I would say to them, hold tight onto your faith, it will see you through, it is the one certain thing that will always be with you, always be there, something from the before that will never be lost. Even when you appear to have lost everything, faith will still be there, in the essence of you, like a perfume always remembered.[1]

IN THE PREVIOUS CHAPTER, I argued that dementia presents us with social, existential, and cultural challenges as persons; and that if we want to find an answer we will have to look more closely at our assumptions about what a human person is. This means that we have to look again at our understanding of what it is to be a human person "before God," our theological anthropology; and we found some fertile resources in the doctrine of humanity in the image of God. However, in order to complete this picture, we need

---

1. Kath Morgan, personal communication in Kevern, "'I Pray That I Will Not Fall,'" 286.

to examine the other side of the coin, our "anthropological theology," how we understand God "before us." Who is the God who is present to us in the midst of this experience of dying "again, and again, and again"? Specifically, how is God present to Kath in her dementia, or accompanying my mother through hers?

The *way* in which God is related to us in the midst of dementia, then, is the point of departure for this chapter; and the question of *who this God is* is the destination we wish to reach. This is a daunting challenge, but fortunately some of the groundwork has been laid by the pastoral theologian Oliver Goldsmith. In a programmatic paper, he examines four possible models as he reflects upon what might constitute the "Good News" to somebody living with dementia. While his primary purpose here is to find something to preach, a comforting word for people with dementia and their families, his exploration of the options helps to flesh out our "anthropological theology" and the issues underlying it.

Goldsmith first outlines a *"Traditional/historical model,"* in which we belong to God by virtue of sharing in the stories that make up the grand sweep of salvation history. The "God of Abraham, Isaac, and Jacob" becomes our God as we recall and recount the stories, are shaped by the narratives; the redemptive work of Christ becomes the route to our redemption as we follow his command to "do this in memory of me." Memory is central as placing us in a shared tradition: we are "held" in God as we make the collective memory of the Church our own, and as we respond to the call to have faith, to reflect, to believe, and to repent. Goldsmith considers, rightly, that this model inevitably progressively excludes those whose memory is vanishing, for "the approach to faith that requires so much memory is problematic for people with dementia."[2]

His second model is one in which all people are called to be *Open to God*, in such a way that, under the influence of the Spirit, "they slowly, imperceptibly almost, move towards the distant horizon of God . . . involved in the gradual divinization of the world." If this is the direction of travel to which God calls us, Goldsmith nevertheless sees it as frequently thwarted by our egos, self-will, and concerns for this world. This means that it requires effort to confront and overcome the impediments we ourselves place in the way so that we may remain open to God's grace. For this reason, he considers it a model that cannot be applied to people living with dementia: it places demands that they are unable to meet, he believes, because "their

---

2. Goldsmith, "Dementia: A Challenge," 129.

world is narrowing, and their egos seem to become more important and dominating as they lose many of their social restraints."[3] This is a curious conclusion, as it seems to leave God unable to move or shape us unless we attain to a sort of perfect openness, and neglects the degree to which all of us are graced despite ourselves. It also seems to reduce our response and openness to the battle to retain our social restraints, which is a very narrow view indeed of our call to discipleship.

Equally curious is his treatment of the *Growth* model, which he describes as the growth from spiritual infancy to a fully mature relationship with God over the course of a lifetime, by analogy with the mundane human life-course. "It is," he says, "as though our spiritual life were a 'dialogue with God' [that] influences and shapes our spiritual growth in the same way that our interaction with other people molds and develops the people that we become." He concludes that this model makes little sense with respect to people with dementia because "their world is diminishing, not opening up . . . . [H]ow do we deal with the experience of dementia in which relationships dwindle, and may be forgotten, and social skills decrease?"[4] This can be understood as a global rejection of the model, inasmuch as it can be applied to all of us who, toward the end of life, can expect to experience diminishment and loss on a range of levels. But, again, it seems too hasty and one-dimensional, as if there is only one way to grow, one mode of relatedness, one language for dialogue with God.

Goldsmith's final approach is via a *Remembered-by-God* model, which he takes to be "the only theological model which seems to encapsulate the 'Good News' for the person with dementia," stressing that "we are remembered by God long before and long after we make any recognizable response to God. We are unconditionally accepted by God, and we are unconditionally acceptable to God." This is the "Good News" that is not dependent on anything we do, believe, or think. For people with dementia and for all of us, the gospel "requires nothing from them, for God has taken all the initiatives and bears all the responsibilities. It is enough for the person just to be . . . ."[5]

The attractions of this last model are clear, and some version of it underlies the majority of pastoral theology developed in response to dementia.[6]

3. Goldsmith, "Dementia: A Challenge," 130.
4. Goldsmith, "Dementia: A Challenge," 130.
5. Goldsmith, "Dementia: A Challenge," 131.
6. See, e.g., Mast, *Second Forgetting*.

It gives a simple and clear message of hope and comfort, both for the individual sufferer and for those close to them, which does not depend upon any doctrinal belief or subtlety beyond the bare affirmation of a present, caring God. This simplicity may be the reason why the slogan "God Never Forgets" seems to crop up repeatedly in the literature.[7] Nevertheless, the model has its limitations both as a theological and a pastoral strategy. There is a tendency to denial of the depth of the questions raised (since although the person forgets, God always remembers) and a profound pessimism (in which dementia is understood only as loss and as a step toward death). But the most serious problem here is that the person disappears as a subject and theological agent. There is nothing for the person to do, no response to be made; they are not being addressed, or challenged, or drawn on the way. They exist only as recipients. For the same reason, this account renders God effectively absent: since Goldsmith does not envision a relationship or (in his words) dialogue between God and the person, God is present only as an abstraction, a guarantor of the eschatological and somewhat vague hope that God will make everything all right in the end.[8] There is a cold irony here: that amid the abandonments and bereavements of dementia, the person is abandoned by and bereaved of the Living God.

These limitations stand out particularly starkly in David Keck's work, *Forgetting Whose We Are: Alzheimer's Disease and the Love of God*, one of the few developed and extensive theological explorations of dementia currently in print. It is a rich book, arising out of his experience of his own mother's dementia, reflected on from a broadly postliberal perspective underpinned by a Barthian theology of the Word. Thus, it treats God's sovereignty as "non-negotiable," focuses on the cross, and takes what it understands to be the traditional body of church doctrine as a given.[9] Although Keck speaks of the suffering Christ, it is as an offering of human suffering to God and not a revelation of a compassionate God. His Christ offers us an "Alzheimer's hermeneutic" in которой the displacement of self entailed in caring for someone with Alzheimer's prepares one for the same

---

7. For example, Ellor, "Celebrating the Human Spirit," 3; Hopkins, "Failing Brain, Faithful God," 37; Atwell et al., *God in Fragments*, 9.

8. Kiblinger, "Theology of Dementia"; Kevern, "What Sort of a God."

9. "I am thankful for doctrine because I believe that only through the faithful transmission of the church's traditional teachings is it possible for me to have hope for my mother; for my father, her primary caregiver; and for the rest of the world which suffers each sunrise and sunset" (Keck, *Forgetting*, 62).

displacement of self in listening for the Word of God.[10] Keck's God is a loving and responsive one, waiting for our openness to the Spirit, but in the final analysis uncompromisingly impassible and sovereign, outside of and above the situation, not within it. His God waits for us, as a loving Father waits for a child, but does not accompany us, as Christ promised to do, "until the end of time."

For some people, this is enough. As we disappear, we are held by God: the deficits we observe are not "dyings" in an absolute sense, but more a sort of "uploading to the cloud" of elements of what we are in God. As we forget, God remembers for us; as we stumble, so we are held in the divine and all-powerful embrace.[11] But stated in this bald way, the God-always-remembers model appears unhelpful because it brackets off the significance of a life actually lived, and with it the prospect of finding meaning in the experience of dementia itself. In the terms laid out in the introduction to this book, it asserts strongly the unchangingness of God in the face of dementia, but in the process it erases the person as a theological subject, along with any real prospect of finding meaning in their dementia. The God thus portrayed is unknowable and unreachable by somebody living with dementia, on the "outside" of the process of change and deterioration, uninvolved in the messy business of living and dying in dementia; waiting at the door, as it were, for it all to be over and the victim to be released into death.

There are, however, more constructive understandings of what it means to say that "God always remembers," and chief of these is John Swinton's subtle and mature treatment of the theme.[12] Swinton treats "remembering" as a transitive verb: in remembering us, God is "re-membering" us, constituting us as human beings in the divine–human relationship. It has little to do with recall of facts or identities, or with the construction of a linear timeline: to be "remembered" is to be accorded an identity, an enduring status. This shift of emphasis enables him to construct a rich pastoral theology. First, he uses it as the basis for theological anthropology itself: we *are* only because we are continually "re-membered" by God, as created and then redeemed beings. "To be held and remembered by God implies some sort of divine action towards the object of the memory. It is

---

10. Keck, *Forgetting*, 227.

11. Goldsmith, "Dementia: A Challenge."

12. John Swinton and I have been discussing these matters for some time. His detailed response to my earlier position on this issue can be found in Swinton, *Dementia*, 198–201.

not purely eschatological action; it is something that happens in the past and the present as well as in the future."[13] It follows, secondly, that our personhood continues as a participation in God's memory since "Human memory is nothing more (and nothing less) than one mode of participation in the memory of God, which is our true memory and our only real source of identity and hope."[14] Thirdly, therefore, the church is called to be a "community of attention" that re-members in solidarity. "The memory of God creates a community of remembering that is called to learn what it means to be attentive to God in those for whom memory is no longer their defining feature or primary learning experience."[15]

Swinton gives us here a rich account of God, as attentive and present to us; of the Church, as God's responsive pastoral agent; and of the person with dementia, as the recipient of these graces. What is still missing from this account, though, is a developed understanding of the person with dementia as theological *subject*, as one whose dementia is not a peripheral accident but part of the medium of a life of discipleship itself, an occasion for challenge and growth toward union with God. The very clarity with which Swinton declares God's constant and sovereign faithfulness leaves little space, it seems, for a positive appreciation of the uncertainties, darkness, and abandonments experienced in dementia. So while his work has been justly praised as a pastoral-theological response to dementia, it leaves God as subject, the person living with dementia as recipient. Their participation in God is through human memory, but this memory is increasingly supplied by the ecclesial community as their own cognitive competence wanes. In defending the honor of a God who does not change as dementia advances, and of a relationship between God and the person that remains constant, he has nevertheless drawn back from according to the experience of dementia itself a theological significance.

We have found that Goldsmith's fourth model leaves us at a dead end because it opens a gulf between God (cognitively competent) and ourselves (progressively cognitively compromised). Rather than painting a picture of a God who is with us in all the circumstances of our life, it asserts God's difference and separateness, leaving us as patients rather than subjects. In passing, we may note the same problem underlies Goldsmith's first model, which he rightly discards as requiring too much of the person with

13. Swinton, *Dementia*, 216.
14. Swinton, *Dementia*, 217.
15. Swinton, *Dementia*, 223.

dementia. Since they do not have the capacity for the complex mental operations required to maintain their place in the tradition, it can only be the collective memory of the Church that "holds" the person in communion with God: neither the individual nor God nor the individual's experience of dementia have any role to play in this process. This does not seem to be the God that Kath is encountering: one who is present to her, although she remains an active agent who can "cloud him out"; one whose love is constant in her anger, who will be there in the core of her being as a "perfume always remembered" even as her memory of her own faith is lost to her. It is not the understanding of God that I would have wanted for my mother, or for myself if dementia lies in my own future. When we talk of the involvement of God in our lives, we are not referring to the remote and disempowering God of either of these models, but a God who is present to us: *Immanuel*.

In the light of this discussion, and in the light of the previous chapter's discussion of the notion of personhood in the image of God, it is worth revisiting the second and third of Goldsmith's models. We should consider whether he has dismissed too lightly the possibility of a living, growing relationship of discipleship and intimacy between God, who is present to us, and the person who is in relationship with this God in the midst of, and maybe even because of, their encounter with dementia. In the twenty-five years since the publication of his discussion of the subject, we have learned much more about the faith of people with dementia, the way it may grow, change, and persist into the later stages of the condition. We are less sure that dementia can simply be described as a succession of deficits or losses and see more clearly the continuing presence of the person with dementia as an active subject. As we shall see later in the book, the language of faith and its expression undoubtedly change; it appears that the character of that faith becomes less rational and verbal, more emotional and intuitive; and that ultimately it may be expressed in a gesture or in simple physicality. But there is no reason to conclude that as a person's dementia progresses they become unable to be open to God or to grow into closer union.

In these two models, characterized as being open to God and as a model of growth, the person is not being "held" as a passive victim, but remains an active theological subject, responsive to the presence of a God who remains present to them as *Immanuel*, God with Us. It is not clear from Goldsmith's original essay in what way he understood these two models to be distinguishable, and for the purposes of this chapter it seems natural to treat them as two facets of the same relationship, in which openness to God results in progress toward true personhood and Christian perfection. The assumption underlying both is that Christian discipleship is not externally imposed on the human person or "against the grain" of their created nature. Instead, it grows out of and develops naturally within the span of a human life, insofar as it is undistorted by sin or concupiscence: it is not progressively denied to a person as a result of their dementia, but they may even be liberated into new patterns of growth as their dementia leaves them more simply open to God. Indeed, we can see this happening in, for example, the testimonies of Bryden and Bute in the previous chapter, or in the signs of growth and deepening uncovered by Tamara Horsburgh in her study of those with early- to mid-stage dementia.[16]

What we are in effect saying here is that people, cognitively impaired or not, grow naturally toward God because of a deep created affinity. This is where the concept of the person as in the image of God, introduced in the previous chapter, comes into its own: for if a person living with dementia continues to be in the image of God, they continue by definition to be open to God; and insofar as they seek to respond to the vision of God revealed in Christ, they grow toward union with God. The presenting question, then, is whether a theological anthropology based on the image of God that includes people with dementia may cast light on what such a growing relationship with God in (and not in spite of) dementia might look like, and what it might say about the God who continues to be present in the midst of it.

Growing into God: From the image of God to the likeness of Christ

In the discussion of the *imago Dei* in the previous chapter, the focus was on our status as *created* in the image of God, based upon the story of our creation in Genesis 1. This was appropriate, because the question to be addressed was about what made us human beings and persons, irrespective of our physical or mental capacities, our social identity or faith commitments. However, it represents only one half of the Christian doctrine of the *imago Dei*: for, according to Paul, if Adam was created in the image of God, then

---

16. Bryden, "Spiritual Journey"; Bute and Morse, *Dementia from the Inside*; Horsburgh, *Impact of Holding Faith*.

Christ is the new Adam in whom that image is perfectly restored and completed in our redemption.[17]

In a startling, staccato summary of the implications of this doctrine of the image, Kilner writes,

> Ultimately, the image of God is Jesus Christ. People are first created and later renewed according to that image. Image involves connection and reflection. Creation in God's image entails a special connection with God and an intended reflection of God. Renewal in God's image entails a more intimate connection with God through Christ and an increasingly actual reflection of God in Christ, to God's glory. This connection with God is the basis of human dignity. This reflection of God is the beauty of human destiny. . . . Christ and humanity, connection and reflection, dignity and destiny—these lie at the heart of what God's image is all about.[18]

When we introduce Christ as the new Adam and the perfect image of God, it changes and completes our theology of the *imago Dei* in some fundamental ways. In the first place, it means that the true image of God is the very presence of God in the world, as Jesus Christ: not an abstract pattern or set of principles to be conformed to, but the substance of a personal encounter.[19] If to be a Christian is to continue to grow, whether with dementia or not, then the direction for that growth is into ever closer union with Christ. Secondly, since the image of God is realized in history, in the life of Jesus of Nazareth, the realization of the image of God in each of us is through the decisions, actions, and relationships that take place in the living of our historical lives. It is here that we encounter Christ, and through Christ the fullness of the Trinity: far from "waiting at the door, as it were," God meets us in the midst of all our circumstances (including dementia) and all can become occasions for the workings of divine grace.

This distinction between our status as created and our call to be active agents in our transformation into the divine image is expressed in a longstanding distinction that was commonplace across the Church until the Middle Ages and continues to be used widely by Eastern Orthodox theologians today: between the divine image (which is ours by virtue of

---

17. See, e.g., Col 1:15; 1 Cor 15:45.
18. Kilner, *Dignity and Destiny*, xi.
19. See the discussion in Crisp, *Word Enfleshed*, 51–70. "Christ is the archetype whose human nature is the blueprint for all other human natures." *Word Enfleshed*, 63.

our createdness) and the divine likeness (into which we grow by the life of discipleship).[20] The point is that there is a sense of *imago* that refers to the being of the individual, and another that refers to a process. We are already shaped in such a way as to receive grace, but grow most completely and faithfully into the likeness of God in Christ when we realize the implications of our relatedness to God in a life faithfully lived, in the way shown to us by Jesus Christ. The distinction will be crucial, particularly when we come to consider late-stage dementia, the point at which many would say that the person who has dementia has already "died inside": for from Comensoli's perspective, there is still a form of discipleship to be realized, a union with God to be sought, and we must attempt to identify it: "To be the kind of creature who is on the way is to be the kind of creature who is in the image of God."[21]

Returning to the two models that Goldsmith rejected—of Openness to God and of Growth in God—I think we can see here a way of making sense of them theologically for someone living with dementia. As Comensoli points out, one of the consequences of the incarnation of Christ, who is the perfect image of God, is that the life which each of us has been given is the one freighted with theological meaning, the stage on which we are offered redemption regardless of our capacities:

> the acceptance of the notion of continuity with regard to creation and redemption means that any human being, by virtue of existing, possesses all that is necessary for being human and is, therefore, redeemable . . . those human beings who have never possessed or who no longer possess certain features that characteristically pertain to human beings, such as agency, are . . . created with all that is proper and necessary to the nature of being human, including the possibility of being redeemed in (but not from) their individual conditions.[22]

This gives the theological backing to the observation made above, that there is no point at which we can clearly say that a person with dementia is

---

20. As Maximus the Confessor puts it, "Every intelligent nature is in the image of God, but only the good and the wise are in His likeness" (quoted in Ware, "Image and Likeness," 56). In the West, the distinction has fallen somewhat out of favor because it rests upon a translation of Genesis 1:27 that is widely held to be mistaken, but it helps to cast light on the distinction Comensoli identifies between two senses of the *imago Dei*. In the remainder of the book, I will use "image" to refer to what Comensoli calls "nearness by likeness" and "likeness" to refer to what he terms "nearness by approach."

21. Comensoli, *In God's Image*, 158. See also p. 210.

22. Comensoli, *In God's Image*, 142.

unable to be open to God or to grow toward God. As well as being created in one sense in the image of God, all of us are given the vocation and the grace through Christ to grow toward union with God through a life faithfully lived, regardless of the circumstances. If this understanding is correct, then it follows that when we seek to grow into the likeness of Christ we are not just trying to be morally good or pretending to be "little Christs" in some sort of theological cosplay: we are responding to a call that grows from our status as in the image of God, expressed by our response to the presence with us of Christ who is himself the perfection of this image. Consequently, we should at least start from the assumption that a person with dementia is able to continue to respond to God, continue to grow toward union, in the midst of their dementia. We should assume that this is the case, because regardless of the extent to which they have lost cognitive capacity, language, physical coordination, and even apparently the ability to respond to their environment in an intentional way, the essentials of a life of discipleship are still in place: the presence to them of Christ, into whose likeness we are called to grow. We must now consider what that phrase, "the presence to them of Christ," entails.

Openness to God: Three bodies of Christ as the different modes of Immanuel in the life of people living with dementia

We grow toward God as we become formed in the likeness of Christ, as a result of our openness to God's call. "Openness to God," in this context, can be understood not just as a vague, passive state of mind but a responsiveness to God that will drive our journey toward union with the divine. This in turn implies that God is available to us and present in our historical lives. So what sort of God is present to us, even in dementia, even when we have no cognitive or mental ability to recall or even recognize who God is? Who is the God who is present in our historical, physical circumstances irrespective of whether our minds are aware of God's presence? The Christian answer has, of course, always been, "Jesus Christ," God incarnate, entering our history and the physical space of the created world, God speaking our language, eating our food, and touching our bodies. The God who is present with us in our own history, whether or not we are aware of it, is present as the body of Christ, inserted into our history.

Surveying the span of salvation history, it seems clear that we can consider Christ as present to us in three distinct ways, represented by three modes of physical presence, the three material, historical "bodies" of Christ. These are represented in Paul's theology in his first letter to the Corinthians:

> So then, whoever eats the bread or drinks the cup of the Lord in an unworthy manner will be guilty of sinning against the body and blood of the Lord. Everyone ought to examine themselves before they eat of the bread and drink from the cup. For those who eat and drink without discerning the body of Christ eat and drink judgment on themselves. That is why many among you are weak and sick, and a number of you have fallen asleep. But if we were more discerning with regard to ourselves, we would not come under such judgment.[23]

In Dale Martin's interpretation, "discerning the body" here entails an understanding of all three senses of Christ's body. First, the broad context is of the Church as the body of Christ, and a failure to discern the body in this sense is manifest in the Corinthians' discriminatory and divisive behavior toward each other. The body of Christ that is the Church brings the presence of Christ into this time and space, and into our collective lives. Christ's future is now tied up with our own: the ways we respond to the promptings of the Spirit and the degree to which we triumph over the challenges and temptations of our age determine the extent to which Christ is manifested to the world in our collective life. There is nothing in this relationship that implies that a person who has dementia, even in its advanced stages, cannot or should not be part of the manifestation of Christ in the present day: the development of dementia in the life of somebody who is a disciple of Christ must be seen as part of the *context* for their discipleship, not the end of it.

Secondly, the immediate context is of the eucharist, and failure to discern the body presumably refers to the way the Corinthians were eating and drinking without reverence for the sacred character of the sacramental meal. Again, there is nothing in this sense of "discerning the body" that implies a certain level of cognitive understanding or theological sophistication, since it has frequently been observed that the work of God in the sacraments is beyond the understanding of all of us, by definition. "Discerning the body" means something different, and presumably is to do with openness to God and to each other in the eucharistic act.

---

23. 1 Cor 11:27–31.

Finally, the warning about being guilty of "sinning against the body and blood of the Lord" can be understood as referencing the historical crucifixion and therefore the fleshly body and blood of Christ in his suffering and death.[24] Christ is present to us in the memory and narrative of the physical, fleshly and historical life of Jesus of Nazareth, culminating in his suffering and death for our redemption as the new Adam and "the firstborn over all creation."[25] This is not just a remembered and narrated presence of Christ: Christ is present in our history, individually and collectively, because God entered the work of time and space; and this is true regardless of whether we remember it consciously or not. Whether we know it or not, the history of the cosmos is stamped in every element with the fact that God has become part of it in Christ.

These three senses of the body of Christ form the basis of Henri de Lubac's extended study of the eucharist and the Church in the Middle Ages, *Corpus Mysticum*, in which he shows how they are woven together in the earliest formulations of the Church and set the pattern for its understanding of the presence of Christ in our midst.[26] One of the striking things about talking of the "bodies" in this way is that they are not theological constructs but *presences*, modes in which, living concrete lives in history, we touch God. In each case, the claim is not just that God can be *thought of* in this way but that God *is in touch* (or was, or will be) with human beings in this mode. We are in the divine image not because we conform to a set of criteria, but because we are in union with Christ as the perfect image of God. We are growing into the likeness of Christ not by completing a cognitive, ethical, or psychological tick-box exercise, but by a process of union through the grace of God. We are no longer hopelessly lost, but have had our status restored as children of God and also as theological agents; not by virtue of possessing a particular set of competencies, but in organic and historical union with Christ.

Each of these ways of understanding Christ's body addresses a distinct question that we need to raise if we are to understand what it is for a Christian who has dementia to grow into union with God, contributing to an understanding of God and God's presence to us in a world of dementia. Each becomes the occasion for and central theme of one of the following chapters, contributing a facet of the account to be drawn together in the

---

24. Martin, *Corinthian Body*, 194–96, cited in McFarland, *Divine Image*, 128–29.
25. 1 Cor 15:45–58; Col 1:15.
26. De Lubac, *Corpus Mysticum*.

concluding section. There is therefore no need to go into detail here, but it may be useful to sketch out the main features by way of an overview.

The suffering and crucified body enables us to reflect on how God is present in our sufferings (including dementia) and what that presence tells us both about God and our calling as in God's image. In history, God took our flesh and so became one with us in all its changes, infirmities, and decompositions: Christ demonstrates that there is no dimension of our fleshliness and mortality, including dementia, that is out of the reach of God. For the same reason, we have the potential to be made into the likeness of God for as long as we are "in the flesh," simply by virtue of being of the same flesh as Christ. This gives us an insight into what shows us the divinity of Christ—the divinity of Christ resides not only in the glorification of his body but also in its deconstruction, not only in the manifestation of his divine personhood but also its apparent erasure on the cross—and, in turn, we may find, paradoxically, that the person living with dementia attains to the likeness of Christ even as the earthly marks of their personhood seem to be being erased.

The ecclesial body opens up the question of how God is encountered in the present, how the body of Christ is realized in the mundane relationships, social networks, and ecclesial institutions that comprise the community of Christians, and how it necessarily is hospitable to "outsiders," particularly in this case people living with dementia. In the ecclesiology developed by Reynolds, the Church becomes the instantiation in history of the image of God to the extent that it finds room within itself for the most vulnerable, and develops a practice of vulnerable openness between all its members.[27] We are ecclesial and theological agents to the extent that we contribute to and challenge the life of the Church, even if this is apparently from outside its formal boundaries and in ways considered contrary to its normal teachings. In chapter 4 I explore this idea through the life of Symeon of Emesa and its interpretation by his fellow Christians, arguing that the Church is manifest, paradoxically, at the point at which it identifies Christ *outside* its institutional boundaries and realizes the ways in which it is *not* the Church.

The sacramental body repeats the same paradoxical pattern, inasmuch as Christ is manifested in *kenosis*, in his concealment under the forms of bread and wine. Similarly, in an enactment of the passion, the grace made manifest through Christ is made available to us at the point of dissolution,

---

27. Reynolds, *Vulnerable Communion*.

as his body is chewed, swallowed, digested. This addresses the question of how we are nourished and restored by God's presence even if we are unable to recognize and respond to it. Once again, God is known paradoxically in the form of a servant, and more than a servant: as a commodity that ceases to exist in the ministration of grace.

In this chapter, I have proposed that we can best think of human beings as persons, as theological subjects, by invoking the theme of the *imago Dei*, meaning that there is an unbreakable relationship with God (maintained by God's unchanging faithfulness) and the call to live faithfully the life that has been given us in history, in the likeness of Christ. In exploring the implications of that claim, we have covered a lot of ground. Starting with a typology of the different ways or models we may use to envision the person living with dementia in relation to God, I have argued, against Goldsmith, that we need to adopt the dynamic models of openness and growth rather than the static claim that "God always remembers" if we are to take seriously the status of people living with dementia as theological subjects. This returns us to a consideration of the image of God, as perfected in Christ, and so introduces Christology as the basis on which we seek to grow into his likeness. In order to understand who we are and where we are journeying we need to consider Christ as present as a body addressing our bodies, providing us with wisdom, belonging, sustenance, and inspiration for the journey.

This discussion has shaped the structure of the remainder of the book. In the next three chapters, I will examine in turn the three "bodies" of Christ which provide us with the living presence of God even in dementia; and which provide us with the template and the context within which we can grow into the likeness of Christ. These explorations will be followed by three chapters that consider what it all may mean for the discipleship of somebody who is living with the progressive changes of dementia, and what their journey in turn tells us about the journey into the transformed life of the kingdom for all of us.

3

Sharing the mind of Christ

My Love, my Light, my Life, do you remember when I was 16 and had a habit of walking to St. Peter's Church in the late afternoons to pray before that larger-than-life crucifix? It depicted you in all your beautiful dark-haired and dark-eyed Jewishness, and it was impossible not to love you to death. One day I was so moved by your predicament on the cross that I had to do something. So I promised that I would always try to hold you up in an effort to prevent your torso from hanging heavily from that cross. I pictured myself doing so through concentrated prayer, willing service, or painful self-sacrifice.

My promise even now calls me to lay down my objections to whatever LBD [Lewy Body Dementia] may do to my body and mind. It cannot destroy my soul. I, who will seem to be lost to LBD, will be found by the one who has earned his title as Savior of the world.[1]

The God who suffers and the physical body of Christ

One of the most influential theological developments of the later twentieth century has been an exploration of God's closeness to us in the life of Christ, and specifically in Christ's sufferings. In this rediscovery of a recurrent theme of Christian piety, the contingency, change, and openness to an uncertain future that mark humanity are not shortcomings, disruptions of

---

1. Hutchinson, "Praying My Way."

true humanity, but are also in the image of God: God is involved with us in all the ups and downs of life lived in history. For Bonhoeffer, it had to be the case because in the twentieth century it seemed to many that the forces of evil were unleashed in such a monstrous way that "only the suffering God could help."[2] Similarly, in the face of the monstrosity of dementia, we may conclude that only the God who experiences dementia can help, and the mode of God's "help" is a revelation of God's deepest nature.

This insight of Bonhoeffer's sets the stage for Jürgen Moltmann's *The Crucified God*, in which he rejects the monolithic assertion of God's impassibility (the doctrine that God, being perfect, can't suffer or change). Taking (and, arguably, misappropriating)[3] Elie Wiesel's account of the three Jewish victims of a hanging by the SS, he develops a Christology that explores how, in Jesus, the whole of God is drawn into the history of suffering and redemption:

> The SS hanged two Jewish men and a youth in front of the whole camp. The men died quickly, but the death throes of the youth lasted for half an hour. "Where is God? Where is he?" someone asked behind me. As the youth still hung in torment for a long time, I heard the man call again, "Where is God now?" And I heard a voice in myself answer: "Where is he? He is here. He is hanging there on the gallows . . . ."[4]

> God does not become an ideal, so that man achieves community with him through constant striving. He humbles himself and takes upon himself the eternal death of the godless and the godforsaken, so that all the godless and the godforsaken can experience communion with him.[5]

---

2. Bonhoeffer, *Letters and Papers*. As Swinton puts it (discussing Bonhoeffer's Christology): "If we are to understand Christ we must understand the relationship of Christ to human beings: the very being of Christ is his being-for-humanity. More, it is impossible to reflect on Christ-in-Christ's self without reflecting on his relationships to humanity. In Christ God creates a space within God's self for human beings; God opens up God's very being to incorporate human beings . . . ." Swinton, "Remembering the Person," 30–31.

3. Rosenbaum, "Elie Wiesel's Secret."

4. Elie Wiesel, quoted by Moltmann in *Crucified God*, 273–74. However, there is some evidence that this is not the version Wiesel wished to be published, and was prevailed upon to "Christianize" it by his French translator, Francois Mauriac. See Rosenbaum, "Elie Wiesel's Secret."

5. Moltmann, *Crucified God*, 276.

God allows himself to be humiliated and crucified in the Son, in order to free the oppressors and the oppressed from oppression and to open up to them the situation of free, sympathetic humanity.[6]

The claim that the story of Jesus's suffering and death on the cross is an act of solidarity between God and suffering humanity has become a commonplace in recent Western theology, and perhaps it is invoked too unthinkingly. As a theological theme, it glosses over some real difficulties with the notion of divine passibility;[7] as a devotional theme it may serve to minimize the reality of suffering in the here-and-now. It is easy to appropriate and "theologize" the suffering of another by claiming that Christ is suffering alongside; easy to smooth the angularity and confusion into an overarching narrative of death and resurrection leading to glorification.[8] The claim that Christ shares in the pain of all suffering people must therefore be made cautiously and meditatively, not to minimize or salve the anguish of the experience but to meet God in it.

Nevertheless, there is something in this story that seems to create in us an intuitive and emotional response; a "rightness" that answers to the sense of overwhelming loss and abandonment that has characterized much of Western experience since the Holocaust; a hope that, somehow, God is present in the midst of it. Although it provides us with no tools to fight oppression and may even contribute to the muting of our response to evil,[9] it gives us a sense that it is worth carrying on in the face of personal experiences of adversity, pain, and suffering. Perhaps for this reason, it has been widely used across a range of theological situations: as Cook comments in relation to dementia, "such places of self-emptying are also places of transcendent encounter, and . . . in Christ we may understand the participation of God in the darkest moments of human experience."[10]

A number of striking and influential works have applied Moltmann's Christology to situations of human suffering, and notably to reflection on

---

6. Moltmann, *Crucified God*, 307.

7. Weinandy, *Does God Suffer?*

8. Indeed, Elie Wiesel himself, in letting his translators "Christianize" his experience, has been criticized for allegedly doing just that, for allowing the trauma of the Holocaust to be domesticated, when it should remain a rage-filled cry of pain. See Rosenbaum, "Elie Wiesel's Secret."

9. I am indebted to my friend Professor Anthony Reddie for making this point to me in the context of Black experiences of oppression.

10. Cook, "Lived Experience," 84.

the meaning and theology of disability. For example, in relation to people with intellectual disability, Stanley Hauerwas (using the language of his time and place) writes, "God's face is the face of the retarded; God's body is the body of the retarded; God's being is that of the retarded."[11] In a similar vein, for Eiesland the resurrection appearances themselves demonstrate God's solidarity with the disabled, for "in presenting his impaired hands and feet to his startled friends, the resurrected Jesus is revealed as the disabled God."[12] Building on Eiesland's work, Reynolds draws out some important dimensions of the *imago Dei*:

> At the cross Jesus subjects himself to disability, and his resurrected body continues to bear the scars as a sign of God's solidarity with humanity. The disabled body of Jesus represents one who understands by embodying disability even in his transformed, resurrected body. . . . Our bodies participate in the *imago Dei* in and through vulnerability and its consequent impairments, not despite them.[13]

Hence,

> Redemption in Christ effects a transformative reversal of the fear-based mistrust we have characterized as the basic impetus to sin. . . . Christ embodies God's self-emptying embrace of creaturely limitation and interdependence, making possible our active openness to God and to others.[14]

> God is in solidarity with humanity at its most fundamental level, in its weakness and brokenness. This is not to romanticize weakness. Rather, here God reveals the divine nature as compassion not only by undergoing or suffering with human vulnerability, but also by raising it up into God's own being.[15]

The conviction that drives Hauerwas, Eiesland, and Reynolds alike is that the "image" in the *imago Dei* is to be taken with the utmost seriousness: to see the person is to see God, and to know God is to know the person. This line of thought enables us to think of the status of a person living with dementia as in the image of God because they reflect the divine nature in their openness and vulnerability toward God. Conversely, we may

11. Hauerwas, *Suffering Presence*, 178.
12. Eiesland, *Disabled God*, 100.
13. Reynolds, *Vulnerable Communion*, 206–7.
14. Reynolds, *Vulnerable Communion*, 197.
15. Reynolds, *Vulnerable Communion*, 18.

encounter a renewed understanding of God's openness and vulnerability in and with the person who has dementia. This is enlightening, but does not quite dispel the image of God "waiting at the door, as it were, for it all to be over and the victim to be released into death," because dementia is not simply an example of suffering in general: it is a particular form of it.

Christ's suffering, our suffering

In traditional Catholic theology, it matters that Jesus did not just suffer but shared in particular sorts of suffering, and the question arises of how, if at all, Jesus shared in something like the experience of dementia. Redemption takes place only because Christ shares in full humanity, and conversely humanity is taken up into divinity. Consequently, an understanding of redemption entails an understanding of what constitutes full humanity, and in particular an understanding of the contribution of human finitude and frailty. So if we want to say that a person who has dementia remains a pilgrim on the journey to union with God; and if we want to say that their dementia is part of that journey and so replete with theological and spiritual meaning; then we must conclude that dementia is also somehow part of the story of the Incarnate Son of God, for as Gregory of Nazianzus pointed out, "what has not been assumed has not been healed."[16]

This process of a two-way reflection between our understanding of God and our experience of personal vulnerability and impairment is part of a well-trodden theological path. Since at least the Middle Ages, the Western Church has taught that, in Jesus, God shared in the sufferings of humanity. Three aspects have been taken as authoritative in Catholic doctrine since Thomas Aquinas, and are generally held to be persuasive in other Christian traditions. First, as noted above, Christ experienced the "defects" intrinsic to humanity, experiencing "the human desires, passions, pains and sorrows both of the body and the soul."[17] Secondly, although he cannot be said to have suffered absolutely every *form* of suffering (because some, such as burning and drowning, are contradictory), he suffered every *kind* of suffering. He endured afflictions from all sorts of people; he endured a "social death" as he was reviled by his enemies and abandoned by his friends; and in his physical body, he endured physical, sensory, and psychological

---

16. McGrath, *Historical Theology*, 46–49.
17. Aquinas, *Summa Theologica*, III 14, III 1.

pain.[18] And finally, Christ's passion was greater than all other pains because of his awareness of the burden of sin he was carrying; from the susceptibility of his soul and body through their perfect constitution; and because he unrestrainedly experienced each of his faculties, so there was no privileged and detached inner sanctum that somehow remained untouched.[19]

Nevertheless, it would be fair to say that many portrayals of Christ's suffering were heroic in nature, stressing his capacity to withstand the pain, and to triumph despite it. It is difficult to see how this could be linked to the suffering of a person with late-stage dementia, when it is difficult to make sense of the concept of intention, let alone fortitude, and some form of passive assent or acceptance is a more realistic spiritual virtue. In this regard, a significant reworking of the narrative of Christ's suffering that departs from the "heroic" portrayal is found in Vanstone's classic work, *The Stature of Waiting*, in which he identifies the heart of the passion as Jesus's being "handed over" in Gethsemane, the hinge between Jesus's life of active ministry and his final calling to powerlessness, voicelessness, and loss. Grace is manifested in Jesus's loss of power, efficacy, and a voice in history, in solidarity with those without agency:

> The passion of Jesus "connects" not simply or even primarily with the human experience of pain: it connects with every experience of passing, suddenly or gradually, into a more dependent phase or area of life.[20]
>
> So when man [sic] waits upon the world—waits even for things so commonplace as food or sunrise or the relief of pain—the image of God is by no means absent from him or imperceptible in him. God also waits; and it is in waiting that He invests the world with the possibility and power of meaning. . . . That man is made, by God's gift, to know and feel his dependence on the world is no less

---

18. "In his head he suffered from the crown of piercing thorns; in his hands and feet, from the fastening of the nails; on his face from the blows and spittle; and from the lashes over his entire body. Moreover, he suffered in all his bodily senses: in touch, by being scourged and nailed; in taste, by being given vinegar and gall to drink; in smell, by being fastened to the gibbet in a place reeking with the stench of corpses, 'which is called Calvary'; in hearing, by being tormented with the cries of blasphemers and scorners; in sight, by beholding the tears of his Mother and of the disciple whom he loved." Aquinas, *Summa Theologica*, III, 46.5.

19. Aquinas, *Summa Theologica*, III 46.6, 7.

20. Vanstone, *Stature of Waiting*, 70.

a mark of God's image in him than that he is made, also by God's gift, to know and feel his capacity for acting and achieving.[21]

The identification between the Christ of the passion and resurrection and people who are relatively powerless, voiceless, or marginalized has become a widely used theological procedure, and similar theological moves are developed in a number of other "theologies of identity."[22] Reynolds extends this as far as including people with hereditary personality disorders, arguing that "at the cross Jesus subjects himself to disability . . . as a sign of God's solidarity with humanity. . . . It suggests that disability indicates not a flawed humanity but a full humanity. Our bodies participate in the *imago Dei* in and through vulnerability and its consequent impairments, not despite them.[23] However, it remains the case that (as far as I know) this procedure has not been extended to the idea of *acquired* cognitive impairment or disability. Occasionally, a connection is made between Christ's sufferings in general and the sufferings of somebody living with dementia, but writers have generally drawn back from ascribing to him the same *kind* of impairment.[24] We have come to recognize that Christ on the cross is stripped of beauty, autonomy, and power, but do not usually see him as stripped of self-awareness.

This lacuna is both predictable and revealing. It is predictable because, as we have already observed, the ideas of "mind" and "spirit" are almost indissolubly linked in the Western Christian tradition, and the idea of God as a sort of transcendent mind is intuitively comfortable in a way that the idea of God as a transcendent body is not. The human spirit is taken to reside in the human mind, which in turn resembles the Divine Mind and is in its image. It is revealing because it helps to explain why we see dementia (literally "loss of mind") as a spiritual challenge of a different order to the loss of physical ability. So if we are to find a place for people living with dementia in the economy of salvation, we must attempt to identify a sense in which Christ shares in the losses of dementia, and in which it is itself

---

21. Vanstone, *Stature of Waiting*, 109, 112.

22. Joh, *Heart of the Cross*; Isherwood, *Fat Jesus*; Douglas, *Black Christ*.

23. Reynolds, *Vulnerable Communion*, 202. Comensoli rejects what he calls the "associating move" because he understands it to make the suffering definitive both for Christ's humanity and that of people with disabilities, and makes a case for a more stringent application of Chalcedonian Christology. However, I do not consider that the two are in the same register, or that the intention of this "associative" move is to redefine divine ontology so much as to open up new understandings of the divine economy.

24. E.g., Morse and Hitchings, *Could It Be Dementia?*, 142–44.

brought within the redeeming ambit of the passion. As Comensoli puts it, "How is someone, in the context of his or her impairment, like Christ in his humanity?"[25] In the following section, we will seek to address this problem.

Christ's delirium, our dementia: Retelling the passion as a site for the "dementia" of Christ

We have established in principle that Christ could have been suffering from a form of cognitive impairment on the cross. It cannot be said that he was experiencing dementia,[26] but the effects of acute delirium are for practical purposes very similar, albeit over a highly condensed time period, and on reflection it seems that the mechanics of crucifixion would have made this virtually inevitable. The clinical reality is that the combined effects of psychological disorientation, sleeplessness, physical shock, dehydration, pain, and injury would in any human being lead to a loss of cognitive function. It is most plausible that, for most if not all of the time that Jesus was on the cross, he was devoid of all agency, cognitive coherence, or a narrative of self-identity,[27] and his cry of abandonment ("My God, My God, why have you forsaken me?") cannot be sanitized away simply as a quotation from Psalm 22. And if Christ can be said to have suffered acute delirium as part of the process of redemption, then acquired cognitive impairments such as dementia are also part of the great sweep of salvation history.

The purpose of this section, then, is to explore what it means to say that, in Christ, God experiences the sufferings of dementia alongside the sufferings of the physical body. The appropriate mode in which to proceed is not so much a critical as a meditative one, seeking (in the mode of the medieval devotionals)[28] to draw the imaginative links between the narrative of the passion and the trajectory of suffering in the individual soul. The two guides who will accompany us on this journey are Elaine Scarry, who in her book *The Body in Pain* offers a detailed study of how torture "unmakes" our individual worlds of meaning by the crushing imposition

---

25. Comensoli, *In God's Image*, 189.

26. Cook rightly points out that "the confusional state associated with severe trauma of this kind would be diagnosed as an acute organic syndrome rather than as a dementia" (Cook, "Lived Experience," 89).

27. Scarry, *Body in Pain*.

28. See e.g., Anselm, *Passion of Christ*

of power; and W. H. Vanstone, whose work considers how that unmaking may, nevertheless, be the road to our redemption.

The premise of this reading of the passion is that redemption is to be found in Jesus's weakness. We must acknowledge from the start that this framing is reading "against the grain" of some elements of the extant narratives, specifically Jesus's words to the penitent thief in Luke and his remarkably composed words to his mother from the cross in John. Clearly if these are taken to be records of Jesus's mental composure after being nailed to the cross, there is no basis for a retelling of the story along the lines I have indicated. But I propose to set them aside as what I believe them to be—theological elaborations or translocations of fragments of the Gospel tradition—and work with a more stripped-down account based largely (though not exclusively) on Mark's account of the passion from Gethsemane through to Calvary. This is the account most explicit about signs of Jesus's weakness and in the opinion of most scholars the one closest to the events themselves: both in terms of time and in preserving an immediacy relatively unfiltered through developing Christological ideas.

The structure is drawn from the themes that comprise the "Sorrowful Mysteries" of the Rosary: the Agony in the Garden; the Scourging; the Crowning with Thorns; the Way of the Cross; and the Crucifixion. It may be objected that to break up the narrative in this way is already to impose an external schema upon it, but it is not an entirely arbitrary one. The current division of the decades of the Rosary has been in use for around six centuries and has structured both the devotional and the dogmatic life of the Church, so it makes clear sense to go with the broad current of Christian wisdom in elaborating the meaning of a dementia-informed reading.

The agony in the garden (Mark 14:32–42)

As already mentioned, Vanstone understands this as the "hinge" of the Gospel narratives, the point at which the activist, miracle-working, teaching, and political Jesus gives way to a "patient": passive, inactive, silent, and swept along by a tide of history over which he attempts to exert no independent agency. It is also perhaps the last point at which we can say that Jesus voluntarily accepted his death (John 10:17–18; Matt 16:21–25). The period in Gethsemane marks the end of Jesus's physical autonomy, although not his psychological agency: he enters the garden voluntarily, but leaves it under guard. He has been placed on a trajectory over which he does not appear to have control. Although he can henceforth influence particular events (e.g., by his replies to Pilate) he cannot determine their overall direction: his condition is now terminal.

In the narrative of Gethsemane, we see Jesus encountering the phenomenon of "social death" that follows on from his passivity, powerlessness, and stigmatized status: his circle of friends and supporters first denies the gravity of the situation (their falling asleep may be seen as a strategy of avoidance) and then flees as the irretrievability of the events becomes undeniable, in a pattern familiar to those experiencing the onset of dementia.[29] At the crucial moment, Jesus is in a hidden place, alone. The only social symbol that is exchanged is that of Judas, a "kiss" whose sign is reversed, a gesture normally of love, here used as one of betrayal. The language of love is itself being degraded in this moment, and so leaves Jesus alone in a way that transcends the simple absence of friends.

As Scarry points out, this is the presupposition and the first consequence of torture. It takes place in hidden places. In the strange world of the torture chamber, the only physical presence, the only potential friend, is the torturer whose role is to betray and whose language corrupts. People who live with dementia know what it is to be left alone, to be isolated by stigma and avoidance, to be trapped in a world of experience that cannot be shared by others, confused by the slippage of language and the inversion of symbols, the loss of friends and confidantes. They also know what it is to lose their autonomy, to be carried away by others and restrained against their will.

The scourging at the pillar (Mark 15:15)

The importance of this episode, dealt with rather cursorily in the Gospels, lies in its concentration on physical insult and injury. As Scarry observes, physical torture isolates us and brings us right back into our bodies: isolates, both because extreme pain cannot be communicated to others; and because at the same time the experience of pain cannot be set at a distance or transcended.[30] It renders everything the same, as everything is consumed in the repetitious, undifferentiated pain. And in the case of Jesus, the pain and the injury is concentrated in the skin: the surface boundary

---

29. Sweeting and Gilhooly, "Social Death"; Ghane et al., "Social Death in Patients."
30. Scarry, *Body in Pain*.

that distinguishes him from others, protects him from dissolution into his surroundings.

Perhaps it is this breaking down of boundaries and distinctions that is itself the most distinctive contribution of the scourging. At the brute physical level, it homogenizes tissues and surfaces, fat and muscle. It (literally) flays the body, destroys the boundary between outside and inside, and lays open its structures right down to the bone. In its repetition, each stroke the same and yet new, it destroys the distinction between past and future in an endlessly iterated present. The notion of an inner core, a "soul" somehow insulated from the events afflicting our bodies, cannot long be maintained in the face of extreme pain that assaults the distinctions between body and soul, inside and outside in a way dramatized in the act of scourging itself: the flaying of the very skin separating us from our environment, tongues of pain crisscrossing the core of his being.

> It is the intense pain that destroys a person's self and world, a destruction experienced spatially as either the contraction of the universe down to the immediate vicinity of the body or as the body swelling to fill the entire universe.[31]

In one sense, the experience of dementia is absolutely isolating in its incommunicability. In another, it destroys the boundaries between self and other, past and present, physical body and "inner self" so that everything starts to dissolve into an undifferentiated mush. Dementia studies have been slow to recognize the essentially *embodied* character of the experience of dementia[32] as Christian thinkers were slow to recognize the essentially embodied character of the incarnation; but here the two meet in a way that we will return to in a later chapter.

The crowning with thorns (Mark 15:16–20)

If the scourging represents the loss of physical boundaries and distinctions, this event is the insult to dignity, to status, and to identity: Jesus has his role returned to him, but in grotesque and parodic form. The crowning continues the inversion of symbols initiated in the kiss of Judas: the sign of glorification is parodied in a theatre of pain and humiliation. It continues

---

31. Scarry, *Body in Pain*, 35.
32. Kontos and Martin, "Embodiment and Dementia"; Eriksen et al., "Experience of Lived Body."

the scourging in the infliction of piercing pain. And it mocks what makes Jesus a king, his powerlessness and silence, for "the goal of the torturer is to make the one, the body, emphatically and crushingly present by destroying it, and to make the other, the voice, absent by destroying it."[33]

The crowning with thorns is "malignant social psychology" at its most vicious and naked: the perverse twisting of Christ's identity as a king into a source of mockery, shame, and physical pain. From a mundane point of view, Christ has utterly failed in the role to which he claimed to be born, in a stripping of role-identity familiar from (for example) Kitwood's "dialectical model" of disabling social interaction;[34] and in this case, it is further symbolized by the thorns, which, dementia-like, reach toward his brain, the seat of his consciousness. When extreme pain is concentrated in the forehead, it becomes impossible to think, to respond, to conceptualize; and in this way, it may be understood to reproduce part of what it is to suffer cognitive impairment.

The way of the cross (Mark 15:21)

As Jesus shoulders his cross and embarks on the *via dolorosa*, for the first time we are back in the world of time, with a progression toward an endpoint. The story also re-emerges from the closed environment of the torture chambers to the quotidian one of people going about their daily business. Following Vanstone, we cannot read too much intentionality or agency in the action of Jesus in carrying his cross. Locked into his own pain, his progress is being driven by others, steered and goaded with blows from those around him: and even in this action he fails, as he stumbles (according to tradition, three times) under the weight of the cross

Unlike in Scarry's analysis (in which all takes place in the enclosed world of the torture chambers), this stage of Jesus's degradation and dehumanization takes place in the public world, and what is being removed is any claim on Jesus's part to dignity or humanity. Despite the social context, the gulf between his (unmediated but incommunicable) pain and the experience of the untortured around him is inconceivable: "The prisoner experiences an annihilating negation so hugely felt throughout his own body

---

33. Scarry, *Body in Pain*, 49.
34. Kitwood, *Dementia Reconsidered*.

that it overflows into the space before his eyes and in his ears and mouth; yet one which is unfelt and unsensed by anybody else."[35]

This is why he is being paraded as a dehumanized symbol of Roman imperial power: as can be the case with a person with dementia, he has been "othered" as an alien, an object of fear or avoidance.[36] But for the first time since the arrest he receives support from others, in the person of Simon of Cyrene (Luke 23:26) and (again, if the tradition is accepted) from Veronica as she wipes his face. The extracanonical story of Veronica takes on a particular power. Recognizing the human identity obscured by blood, pain, and confusion, she wipes his face, literally restoring a face to him. Subverting the narrative of power in which he has been subsumed, she restores to him a social presence. As Jesus's inner world collapses, so others take up responsibility for supporting his self-narrative, and the fulfillment of Jesus's calling thus becomes dependent on the activities of others.

The crucifixion (Mark 15:22–39)

As Jesus hangs on the cross, the divestment of his self as we typically understand it (as a cognitive center, with autonomy, intentional agency, social status, and ordered movement through time) is complete. All that is left to him now is a repeated, pointless lifting of his body against the tearing pain of the nails, in order to take the next breath. Insofar as we believe Jesus to be truly human, it is certain the combination of pain, abandonment, dehydration, and depersonalization will have left him in a state of acute delirium, at best intermittently aware of his surroundings.[37] In Scarry's terms, his "Unmaking" is complete. As we have seen, there has been a violation of boundaries on several levels: the destruction of the skin, the invasion of the psyche, the loss of individual subjectivity. The only "separateness" left to Jesus is the physical distancing in space afforded by the cross itself.

Indeed, for Vanstone, the passion narrative is, to all intents and purposes, over at this point, as he maintains that it is Jesus's assent to the "handing over" in Gethsemane and his continued compliance from that point forward that comprise the work of redemption. He argues that the focus on the cross leads us to emphasize the centrality of Jesus's physical death as the decisive moment in the narrative: an emphasis that he considers misplaced:

35. Scarry, *Body in Pain*, 36.
36. Doyle and Rubinstein, "Person-Centered Dementia Care."
37. Habermas, Kopel, and Shaw, "Medical Views."

"If we say that Jesus was 'handed over unto death' we do not necessarily mean that He was handed over in order that He might be killed: we mean that He was so totally, so unreservedly, handed over that the ultimate possibility that He would be killed was not excluded."[38] So instead of focusing on the moment of death, he lingers on the ways in which (in the words of the advertisement with which we began chapter 1), Jesus has already died "again, and again, and again."[39]

Who is the Christ who suffers? Dementia, delirium, and redemption

Throughout the course of the meditation above, connections have been made between the passion narrative and elements of the experience of living with dementia. Reflecting on von Balthasar's analysis of the death of Christ, James and Stevens comment,

> In becoming passive, Jesus embodies the character of a frailer or older person often enacted in the process of dementia. The dementia sufferer almost becomes an object about whom decisions are made, actions are "done" to them, and many will fear both the societal stigma around the loss of control and the unknown. . . . Jesus, in a parallel manner, underwent the experience of others stripping away his capacities and decisions being made that had a profound impact on his body and mind and thus placed himself in solidarity with the human experience of ageing and dying.[40]

To what extent, though, could it be said that Jesus "shared the sufferings" of dementia? Some clarity may be found by reviewing what Scarry presents as the eight characteristics of extreme pain as revealed in her study of torture:[41]

1. Its "extreme aversiveness . . . a pure physical experience of negation"

---

38. Vanstone, *Stature of Waiting*, 78.
39. Vanstone, *Stature of Waiting*, 79–87.
40. James and Stevens, "Behold, the Human Being," 105. Following von Balthasar, they consider the abandonment by God to continue into and be intensified on Holy Saturday, but this is a contested interpretation of the events after Jesus's death (see e.g., Oakes, "Internal Logic") and will not be elaborated here.
41. Scarry, *Body in Pain*, 52–56.

2. and 3. The "double experience of agency": it seems to be, at the same time, something that our own body is doing to itself and something alien arriving from outside

4. An "almost obscene conflation of the private and public" as the shameful failures of the intimate body are exposed for others to see and comment on in the social space

5. Its ability to destroy language: "Eventually the pain so deepens that the coherence of complaint is displaced by the sounds anterior to learned language"

6. "The obliteration of the contents of consciousness. Pain annihilates not only the contents of complex thought and emotion but also the objects of the most elemental acts of perception"

7. Pain's totality, spanning inside and outside to destroy anything "that is alien to itself and threatening to its claims"

8. Its resistance to objectification: indisputably real to the sufferer, but unreal to others unless labeled with a diagnosis

This list puts a framework around the narrative of the passion as above, but also around the narrative of dementia: it should be apparent by now that all of these features to some extent define how dementia is experienced and responded to. Although we will never be able to reconstruct Jesus's sufferings and state of mind with any certainty, there is enough here to establish a congruence between the elements of the crucifixion narrative and the losses associated with the progress of dementia.

It can be said with some confidence that, in his passion, Jesus shared in the sufferings of somebody on the journey through dementia. However, at the same time this account seems to remove the redemptive significance of the passion, for everything that identifies Jesus as the Christ appears to have been obliterated in the tortures he has undergone. If we can answer the question "What maintains the identity of Christ in his acute delirium?" it will lead us toward an answer to two others: "What does it mean to say that Christ is present to the person in the midst of their dementia?" and "What does it mean to say that the person living with dementia remains, nevertheless, present to Christ?" There are two insights that arise from the discussion in this chapter that may provide some fertile food for thought:

The first is that *the identity of Christ is not negated by his delirium, but reasserted*. Since dementia is a possibility intrinsic to the condition of being human, when we develop dementia we become more visibly human, rather than less so, in the sense that another of the possibilities intrinsic in the human condition is made visible in us. In the terms laid out by Comensoli (see chapter 2) Christ is the perfect image of God in his embrace of the form of life God prepared for him; and we are formed in the image of Christ if, should we be called to it, we assent to the dementia prepared for us.

It may be objected that what is striking in the passion narrative is how the identity of Christ is, by all mundane standards, being progressively stripped from him. However, there is a revealing twist to this account. Paradoxically, it is when Christ "loses his identity" on the cross, that we know him for who he truly is, as the perfect expression of the self-emptying God. Perhaps some of this is caught in the exclamation of the centurion in Mark, that "Truly this was [the] Son of God!"[42] Analogously, if we want to say that, even at the point of greatest forgetfulness of God and of self we encounter God, then it is important to say that God is present in that very moment: not as over-against our forgetfulness, but *in* and *through* it. Counterintuitively, we are led toward the conclusion that in the absences and deficits of dementia there may be opening a way to us for true intimacy with the Christ whose identity is known only in his surrender. Thus, the assertion that Christ also suffered similarly on the cross opens the way for an understanding of dementia as potentially grace-filled; as potentially an agent for union with God rather than estrangement from God. This, perhaps, is an answer to Keck's declaration that dementia is an evil because it is "Deconstruction incarnate."[43] Christ is "the Incarnate who undergoes deconstruction," and the good news may be that, as a result, we encounter the Incarnate in our deconstruction. In the words of Reynolds, "This vision is paradoxical and subversive. More than simply idealizing vulnerability, it produces what I have called a 'metaphorical reversal' that exposes the false pretenses of the cult of normalcy and opens up the possibility of living in light of God's love. And such love is presented redemptively in the person and work of Jesus Christ."[44]

---

42. Surprisingly, Scarry comes to a similar conclusion when considering the cross: "It is not that the concept of power is eliminated, and it is certainly not that the idea of suffering is eliminated. They are no longer manifestations of each other: one person's pain is not the sign of another's power. The greatness of human vulnerability is not the greatness of divine invulnerability. They are unrelated and therefore can occur together: God is both omnipotent and in pain." Scarry, *Body in Pain*, 214.

43. Keck, *Forgetting*, 32.

44. Reynolds, *Vulnerable Communion*, 176.

The second point is that *human identity and awareness is held corporately*. If human identity and autonomy has a narrative shape, that does not imply that the narrative of the individual is solely the concern of that individual. On the contrary, the story that comprises one's "identity" in time and space is the product of a collaborative effort, a negotiation between self and others.[45] Thus, ironically, it is at the point at which they are unable to offer him any support, at the foot of the cross, that the friends and family who deserted him at Gethsemane have returned, to gather there. Those who abandoned him at the end of his life return to take his body from the cross, protect it from the scavengers:

> while he was then "forgotten" by human institutions and authorities, and even while Son and Father experienced alienation, his body was taken down from the cross, cared for and laid to rest in the tomb. Normal practice was for such a body to remain on the cross to be food for scavenging animals or to be dismembered, but there was someone to prevent this, someone to remember and re-member, even in the utter desolation that was Golgotha. Joseph and Nicodemus were re-membering Jesus, giving care and embracing his identity as an embodied human being in the same way that carers re-member the identities of those they love who have dementia.[46]

These are the historical individuals who form a chain of touch from the physical body to the nascent Church, the ecclesial body. They are the ones who must carry the narrative forward over the coming three days and witness to its culmination in the resurrection. We may say that the anamnesis at the heart of the eucharist, the "re-membering" that constitutes the central act of the Church, is already taking place at the cross: Christ's death already involves the community that will commemorate and celebrate it as the relatives and disciples gather at its foot. Analogously, in the life course of somebody living with dementia, progressively more of the burden of narration may be taken by those around them—the second-person and third-person perspectives—and less by the subject; but this is not to degrade the narrative or the subject of it. In a social context, a person may persist as a person even if they are individually unaware of the fact.

Translated into a theological context, these lines of thought suggest a way to talk of how the work of redemption apparently goes forward without

---

45. Radden and Fordyce, "Into the Darkness."
46. James and Stevens, "Behold, the Human Being," 106.

Jesus's conscious participation; and the work of our "attaining to the whole measure of the fullness of Christ"[47] continues whether or not we are able consciously and intentionally to participate in the process. Christ and the Christian disciple who has dementia continue to draw close, to dwell in each other, regardless of (or in some senses because of) the loss of a conscious, intentional "personal identity": in their shared experience, in their graced histories, and in the work of "active, collaborative authorship of the self-narrative" continued in the graced community surrounding both.

It is this latter aspect that will inform the two chapters that follow: an "ecclesiological turn" as I develop the argument that the narrative connecting Christ and people who have dementia may be "held" by the community of people committed to both. One immediate consequence of this line of thought is that there is no longer a clear line to be drawn between the work of Jesus on the cross and the work of the embryonic Church in remembering and witnessing to it: indeed, the two can be considered two expressions of the same body, as "the Church was born from the side of our Savior on the Cross like a new Eve, mother of all the living."[48] We may say that the work and identity of Christ "leaks" into that of the early Church.[49]

Traditionally, it is this Church which has shouldered the responsibility of maintaining the stability of Christ's memory in its scriptures, its rituals, its polity, and its disciplines: policing to ensure clear boundaries and consistent administration. However, our consideration of the work of Christ in relation to its members with dementia suggests that there may be another dynamic at work in the bodies of Christ, one in which, paradoxically, Christ is manifest through unknowing, loss of definition and "identity," transgression of the clear binaries that create good order. The next challenge is to locate the continuing presence of this "deconstructed" Christ and the people who, like him, do not "make sense" in the accepted understanding, in relation to the actual, historical communities of Christians who bear his name. How do people with dementia fit into the life of the churches, and how do they need to respond in order to manifest the presence of Christ in his body the Church? Might it be that the historical churches, too, are in regular need of a sort of dementia, an invasion of unreason, in order to save them from their own "hypercognitive" state?

---

47. Eph 4:13.
48. Pope Pius XII, *Mystici Corporis*, §28.
49. Moltmann-Wendel, "Feminist Theology."

4

Symeon of Emesa and the "holy fools" of God

The manner of his entry into the city was as follows: When the famous Symeon found a dead dog on a dunghill outside the city, he loosened the rope belt he was wearing, and tied it to the dog's foot. He dragged the dog as he ran and entered the gate, where there was a children's school nearby. When the children saw him, they began to cry, "Hey, a crazy abba!" And they set about to run after him and box him on the ears.

On the next day, which was Sunday, he took nuts, and entering the church at the beginning of the liturgy, he threw the nuts and put out the candles. When they hurried to run after him, he went up to the pulpit, and from there he pelted the women with nuts. With great trouble, they chased after him, and while he was going out, he overturned the tables of the pastry chefs, who (nearly) beat him to death. Seeing himself crushed by the blows, he said to himself, "Poor Symeon, if things like this keep happening, you won't live for a week in these people's hands."[1]

---

1. Krueger, *Symeon*, 45–46.

Locating the ecclesial body of Christ in a time of dementia

People with dementia can appear to church communities as a disruption, a disturbing "other" whose behavior or communication presents a challenge to their calm weekly rhythms in a way not unlike the appearance of Symeon of Emesa in the passage above. In this chapter, I will explore the role and contribution of people with dementia to the life and identity of the Church by reflecting on Symeon's story, and bringing it into a conversation with some lines of thought regarding the Church from theologians of disability.

In the light of chapter 3, we start with the suffering, fleshly body of Christ whose physical identity was tortured and "deconstructed" to the point of erasure in his passion, that at this point gives birth to the community that somehow makes up the body of Christ through history. The physical, fleshly body of Christ opens out to become the Church at Calvary, when the people who comprise the seed of the future Church gather around his cross at his death: "it was on the tree of the Cross, finally, that He entered into possession of His Church, that is, of all the members of His Mystical Body."[2] But in another sense, the fleshly and ecclesial bodies of Christ may be understood as always already united in the purposes of God: in a striking image from the papal encyclical *Mystici Corporis Christi* we read that "hardly was He conceived in the womb of the Mother of God, when He began to enjoy the Beatific Vision, and in that vision all the members of His Mystical Body were continually and unceasingly present to Him, and He embraced them with His redeeming love. . . . In the crib, on the Cross, in the unending glory of the Father, Christ has all the members of the Church present before Him and united to Him."[3]

If at Calvary the body of Christ that is the Church takes on a historical existence, the earthly church must still work to realize its true vocation to be "as it were, the filling out and the complement of the Redeemer, while Christ in a sense attains through the Church a fulness in all things."[4] This means that the earthly, historical church is two things at once. Theologically, "the Church marks the locus of Christ's objective presence in the world . . . . Insofar as the Church is specifically Christ's body, he is the source of

---

2. Pope Pius XII, *Mystici Corporis*, §30.
3. Pope Pius XII, *Mystici Corporis*, §75.
4. Pope Pius XII, *Mystici Corporis*, §77.

its identity."[5] Sociohistorically, the community that claims to be the Church has yet to be fully realized: although "Christians derive their identity from this particular human life . . . the full shape of this life is inseparable from the total number of those who are now part of his story."[6] The Church is presently on pilgrimage, anticipating but yet to fully express its final eschatological perfection, and this will only be fully manifest when all those who make up its members are recognized and treated as such.[7] Clearly, "the total number of those who are now part of his story" includes people living with dementia, many of whom will have a record of faithful Christian discipleship and church membership stretching back decades, and the Church only realizes its true identity when it includes these members as well. When in our churches we seek to include, support, and nurture the faith of people in our community who are showing symptoms of dementia, we are not only demonstrating our pastoral concern and being compassionate to those in need; we are also making present in this time and place the body of Christ and participating in the transformation of the community from a mundane collectivity of secular individuals into the Church.

However, the presence of hitherto faithful and admirable church members who are living with dementia presents real challenges to many commonly held assumptions about the character of church life. Some of the common symptoms—apparent changes in behavior, personality, and conviction—may call into question the person's credentials as a member of the community of believers at all. People whose qualities have satisfied the most demanding criteria for church membership—deep understanding, correct doctrine, unwavering commitment, and unimpeachable behavior—may appear to change inexorably into someone else, before the eyes of their community. This is particularly pronounced in the case of Frontal Lobe Dementia, in which social inhibitions and impulse control are among the first functions to be impaired while memory, coordination, and cognitive ability may be preserved for much longer, leading often to unpredictable and disruptive behavior. Such behavior may appear to be less like a loss of capacity and more like the sort of sinfulness the church seeks to exclude: sexual disinhibition, unacceptable language, blasphemy, potential violence.

Perhaps the most natural response is to treat the potentially disruptive and challenging presence of members living with dementia as a pastoral

5. McFarland, *Divine Image*, 56.
6. McFarland, *Divine Image*, 54.
7. Pope Paul VI, *Lumen Gentium*, §48.

issue, a practical problem to be solved in such a way that the church demonstrates its compassion to the "outsider," welcomes the "stranger." As I mentioned in chapter 2, there is a significant body of Christian writing about dementia along these lines, which has yielded a rich seam of practical and pastoral advice for church ministers and their congregations about how they should respond. However, most of this material does not reach further into the issues to consider the significance of people living with dementia for the very existence and identity of the Church; what their presence contributes positively to the health of our communities or why the Church needs them if it is to flourish. We need to ask a wider question: "Granted that the saints and the poor are characterized by a relationship of utter dependence on God that makes them uniquely transparent to Christ, in what sense, if any, is the Church dependent on them?"[8] In the following sections, I will explore this question through the narrative *Life of Symeon of Emesa*, and consider what such an ecclesiology of "the other" may have to tell us.

Enter the holy fool

Within the Church, there is a long and at times inspiring tradition that considers the place and role in it of people with congenital cognitive disabilities. However, there is no such tradition of thinking about people with acquired and progressive cognitive conditions and, as I said earlier, they present a rather different set of issues. Dementia was much less common until the significant increases in life expectancy of the last hundred years, and the distinctions between folly, dementia, mental illness, and disability only became widely established in the West from the Renaissance onward.[9] This means that we must look to other traditions for inspiration regarding how people with progressive, late-onset intellectual and behavioral issues might be understood and acknowledged in the church. The one I have selected here for further study and reflection is the "holy fool" tradition,[10] which has been largely developed by Eastern Orthodox Christianity,[11] but

---

8. McFarland, *Divine Image*, 82.
9. Yong, *Theology and Down Syndrome*, 28.
10. I am indebted to Dr. Ralph Norman for pointing out this parallel.
11. For a contemporary Russian example, see Sergey Korsakov's 2006 film, *The Island*, available to view on YouTube at https://www.youtube.com/watch?v=Wz-vegualMg.

which continues to exert a quiet influence in the West.[12] Such "holy fools" are always marginal to the ecclesial societies in which they find themselves. They are disruptive and sometimes obscene, and in this respect may provide an echo of the presence in our churches of some people who have dementia. But they were also counted holy by the Church, and I shall argue that the reasons for this present some challenges to our own ecclesiology.

My proposal to compare dementia to the holy fool tradition may have given rise in the reader to a queasy sense that actually they do not belong together. What might be the source of this aversion, and what might it tell us about the assumptions we bring to dementia in the Church? It seems to me worth exploring the following facets of my own reaction. First, there is the juxtaposition of the word "fool" with a discussion of those who are living with dementia and otherwise mentally different, which raises individual and corporate memories of marginalization and socially imposed rejection. Although we may claim to value the contribution of the "disheveled, gauche, tragic-comic figure of the fool,"[13] such a person is unlikely to be welcomed into our pulpits or pastoral teams. Talk of fools thus sharpens the question of what, if anything, a person living with dementia has to offer to the Church, and whether foolishness is a gift we wish to receive.

Secondly, the use of the term "holy" in relation to dementia seems to ignore the fact that many people with dementia, as their condition progresses, behave in ways that are superficially very *unholy*: they can be profane, disruptive, violent, promiscuous, and heretical. When such behavior is recorded in the holy fool tradition, it is generally as "pretending to madness." But no such claims are made for those who are living with dementia, and it is a long step from the holy fool to celebrating the holiness of a church member whose dementia manifests in disruptive behavior. How is the church community supposed to discern holiness in madness? What happens to normal church life when these two categories are confused?[14]

---

12. This is particularly visible in the continuing appeal of Francis of Assisi, but may also be seen in, for example, early Methodism or the "simple souls" of Protestant pietism.

13. This is one of the models offered by Campbell, *Rediscovering Pastoral Care*, 47.

14. As Michel de Certeau writes in his discussion of the fourth-century story of the "Idiot Woman" from the *Lausiac History*, "The passage in *Lausiac History* that introduces the first idiot woman was later entitled 'She who simulated madness.' The title, and the first sentence from which it was taken, dispose too quickly of an unresolvable question: Is the madness real or affected? Or real because affected? Or made up of several kinds of madness?" Certeau, *Mystic Fable Volume 1*, 32.

Finally, and as a result of this deliberate confusion of categories, there arise some disturbing questions about the operation of grace. The holy fool tradition suggests that grace operates by interrupting the life of the church, instead of (or perhaps as well as) operating through its regular institutional activities, and this interruption occurs regardless of intellectual justification or foresight. It suggests that chaos and disruption may be part of that grace and that its contemporary expression may include those members who are living with dementia. It is perhaps uncomfortable for settled Christian churches in a time of social stability to have to contemplate this possibility. What changes would have to take place in order for graced chaos to be welcome?

The particular example I will now use to develop these themes is Leontius's *Life of Symeon the Holy Fool*.[15] This was arguably the most influential text on the subject, inspiring as it did a pattern of devotion and imitation across the entire Mediterranean world, and touches on something that looks like dementia. In the opinion of John Saward some holy fools were genuinely mentally disturbed, although this does not undermine their contribution;[16] and Symeon's combination of disinhibition with apparently unimpaired intellectual and physical capacity is certainly suggestive of Frontal Lobe Dementia.[17] What is remarkable here is that although he was clearly rejected by many of those with whom he came into contact, the Church ultimately came not only to accept but to revere his contribution.

Symeon died around 590, and the *Life of Symeon the Holy Fool* by the renowned hagiographer Leontius, bishop of Neapolis in Cyprus, was probably written around fifty years later. It circulated widely and became the pattern for a whole genre of subsequent stories, which fed a popular cult.[18] Leontius's *Life* begins by following the standard hagiographies of the desert saints in, as Roger Scott has put it, "a dull narrative full of prayers, visions and platitudinous acts of piety."[19] Symeon grows up in a city (Edessa) but leaves it with his companion and witness, John, to seek perfection in a desert monastery and then as a hermit for a total of twenty-nine years.

---

15. Krueger, *Symeon*. Extracts are taken from his translation of the life, with page numbers as indicated.

16. Saward, *Perfect Fools*, 26.

17. See, e.g., Alzheimer's Society, "Caring for My Dad with Frontotemporal Dementia."

18. Saward, *Perfect Fools*, 19–20.

19. Scott, Review of *Symeon the Holy Fool*.

However, both the style and content of the *Life* take on a racier tone when Symeon (for unspecified reasons) leaves the desert to continue his search for sanctity in a return to the city. He enters Emesa as a stranger, both in the sense that he is not known there and in the sense that he comes from the desert, the strange place that represents wildness, peril, and the abode of demons. He is the very definition of an "outsider."

Symeon's alien character is reinforced by his behavior, which would be considered aberrant and eccentric in any society. In addition to the incidents reported in the short section at the head of this chapter, a long catalogue is given of socially disruptive actions. He defecated in the street, wandered around naked, entered the women's section of the bath-house and pretended to attempt to rape a woman.[20] This was enough to mark him down as the "Crazy Abba." His behavior is variously interpreted as that of a fool, a rogue, and a holy man with divine powers, and a number of the incidents recounted depend for their dramatic effect on the debate they provoke among the onlookers regarding his character. They read his behavior in two divergent ways: as a form of "madness" or as a form of holiness that, in its prophetic force and rejection of superficial norms, appeared in the form of madness.

Leontius writes,

> the saint wanted to destroy his edification, so that the tavern keeper would not expose him. One day when the tavern keeper's wife was asleep alone and the tavern keeper was selling wine, Abba Symeon approached her and pretended to undress. The woman screamed, and when her husband came in, she said to him, "Throw this thrice cursed man out! He wanted to rape me." And punching him with his fists, he carried him out of the shop and into the icy cold. Now there was a mighty storm and it was raining. And from that moment, not only did the tavern keeper think that he was beside himself, but if he heard someone else saying, "Perhaps Abba Symeon pretends to be like this," immediately he answered, "He is completely possessed. I know, and no one can persuade me otherwise. He tried to rape my wife. And he eats meat as if he's godless."[21]

> He played all sorts of roles foolish and indecent, but language is not sufficient to paint a portrait of his doings. For sometimes he pretended to have a limp, sometimes he jumped around,

---

20. Krueger, *Symeon*, 148–49.
21. Krueger, *Symeon*, 147–48.

sometimes he dragged himself along on his buttocks, sometimes he stuck out his foot for someone running and tripped him. Other times when there was a new moon, he looked at the sky and fell down and thrashed about. Sometimes also he pretended to babble, for he said that of all semblances, this one is most fitting and most useful to those who simulate folly for the sake of Christ.[22]

This clash of interpretations structures and shapes the whole text of Leontius's *Life*. The whole narrative aims to unsettle conventional images of sanctity, as it repeatedly inverts and then restores conventional notions of good and bad. Symeon appears bad, but is good; respectable Christian society appears good, but is blind and ignorant. We are required to choose between the perspective of the "fleshly" (who are misled by the surface appearance of Symeon) and the attitude of his spiritual friend and companion, the Deacon John, who sees through the strange behavior to its motive. It is John's interpretation and testimony that forms the basis for Leontius's biography.[23] Symeon, he claims, is much more venerable than most because he rose to the most pure and impassible height, although to those more impassioned and more fleshly he seemed to be a defilement, a sort of poison, and an impediment to the virtuous life on account of his appearance. Because of these things he was most pure, just as a pearl which has traveled through slime unsullied. Indeed, I say that through spending time in the city, hanging around with women, and the rest of the deception of his life, he truly sought to show a weakness in the virtuous life to the slothful and pretentious and the power granted by God to those who truly serve against the spirits of evil with all their souls.[24]

It should be obvious by now that a key element of this text is its dialectical structure. Symeon is outside the normal boundaries of the church, socially, morally, and behaviorally.[25] In the eyes of the "fleshly," the conven-

22. Krueger, *Symeon*, 155–56.

23. According to Leontius, "This aforementioned John, beloved of God, a virtuous deacon, narrated for us almost the entire life of that most wise one, calling on the Lord as witness to his story, that he had written nothing to add to the narrative, but rather that since that time he had forgotten most things." Krueger, *Symeon*, 125.

24. Krueger, *Symeon*, 122.

25. "His daily provocative and shameless acts usually took place in the market, the centre of the city's social life, so that they could always be witnessed by the widest possible audience. He violated church rules by publicly eating meat during the Holy Week. He danced in the streets, tripped passers-by and pretended to have seizures. He associated with outcasts, such as the possessed, whom society treated with great cruelty. He spent his time with actors, whose occupation was considered immoral, and visited prostitutes,

tional church members of urban Emesa, Symeon appears as the quintessential outsider, blowing in from the desert: "mad" or sinful; destructive; lazy and weak in comparison with their own life as sane, moderate, constructive, industrious, and powerful urbanites. He threatens to disrupt and destroy their settled and respectable church life. Not so, says Leontius: benefiting from the spiritual perception of John, we can see that his apparent madness is holiness; his acts of disruption, prophetic gestures; his slothfulness a challenge to the materialist urbanites and his apparent weakness a vulnerability born of abandonment to God. From the perspective of the coming kingdom of God, it is the churchpeople of Emesa who are the "outsiders." They are suffering from a sort of madness in their refusal to listen; self-destructive in their waywardness; lost in their slothful complacency and perilously weak in their faith. The more rigid their response to him and the fiercer their disapproval, the more extreme must his behavior become in an attempt to puncture their complacency. But the more extreme his behavior, the more the fleshly become scandalized and resistant to change.[26] The earthly church succumbs, as Reynolds points out in relation to disability, to basic social drives:

> The human need for orientation and belonging wields a mighty yet corruptible power. When endangered, it can manifest itself collectively in protective strategies that aim to secure and fortify communal stability. For the different and the "other" disorientates the familiar, threatening to undo the trust we have placed in its conventions. So . . . borders are ossified and made accessible only to those whose body capital amounts to an exchangeable value.[27]

So by a dizzying set of inversions, we find the world turned upside down. The boundaries of the Byzantine church of Emesa are not containing and protecting the ecclesial body of Christ, but excluding it; indeed, there may be in Symeon's actions a parodic echo of some of Jesus's own.[28] The

---

calling them his 'friends.' Respectable citizens were scandalized, ignoring the fact that despite his provocative frequenting of brothels and taverns, he remained chaste, pure, unmoved by carnal temptations, having conquered the desirable apathy." Poulakou-Rebelakou et al., "Holy Fools," 98.

26. As Saward points out, the "holy fool" is a troubling of a flourishing and peaceful church, and has no place in turbulent times. See Saward, *Perfect Fools*, 28.

27. Reynolds, *Vulnerable Communion*, 59.

28. Krueger points out that a number of his actions are variations on incidents in the life of Christ, e.g., entering the city with a dead dog rather than a donkey. See Krueger, "Comedy to Martyrdom."

Spirit that is supposed to inspire it blows where it wills, outside the city walls. Leontius's message seems to be that, in seeking to define and preserve the body of Christ by excluding the apparently insane, the unmanageable, and chaotic, we suffocate it by excluding the Spirit. Indeed, by the time Leontius is writing his hagiography, Emesa had fallen to a Muslim army and part of its most important church building, the Church of St. John, had been converted into a mosque. For Leontius, then, there was potentially a graphic representation of what happened to a church when it excludes the transgressive Spirit from within its protected boundaries: it ceases to be the Church at all, and the body of Christ remains outside its definitions.

The hermeneutics of the holy fool and the boundaries of the body of Christ

In Leontius's hagiography, it at first appears we are being told the story of someone who is mad. However, they seem to be mad only because their society is mad. Deluded by phantoms and blinded by attachments, the church community at Emesa was a place of "malignant social psychology." It was because of their own mental or spiritual illness that they could not perceive the true character of the person behind the deeds. Like the fleshly in the presence of the holy fool, we too must reckon with the possibility that the dementia lies with us as well as them; that a hermeneutical choice to take people with conditions such as dementia seriously is a precondition of both our own mental or spiritual health and our understanding of it in others.

That said, Leontius offers us some sort of resolution of the dialectic, so there is the possibility of conversion. Once the hermeneutic choice is made by the reader to take Symeon with full seriousness, the nature of society's madness becomes clear and transformation can take place. If the earthly church abandons its fleshly respectability, its excluding norms, and its identifying boundaries to embrace all those who enter it, whether dragging a dead dog or throwing nuts, it has the potential to be healed. Paradoxically, the Church becomes recognizable as the ecclesial body of Christ at the point at which its boundaries dissolve and its life overspills its neatly defined identity. If we are neither holy fools nor the fleshly, then we can understand and profit from this story.

As I have already noted, there is something queasy about identifying Church members who live with dementia with the tradition of the "holy fool," not least because we want the Church to be inclusive and such language seems already "othering." But on the other hand, it would be dishonest to pretend that a person undergoing some of the behavioral and social changes characteristic particularly of Frontal Lobe Dementia is going to be treated as if their status in the ecclesial community has not changed, and as if all that is required of the church is increased pastoral support: indeed, such a claim would itself be to erase the experience of the condition and the status of the person living with it in favor of a generic "caring" response. It is both more honest and more constructive to accept that people are integrated into the Church in different ways, and that there is a sort of dialectic at work in our encounter with and response to people who do not fit our norms, one that resembles the relationship between the people of Emesa and Symeon, but also Kitwood's dialectical model of dementia.[29] We are called not to erase the difference, but to work through it for our own conversion also.

So how might we collectively respond to a church member whose dementia is such that they do not communicate in the agreed ways, and who disrupts the normal life of the community? By analogy with the *Life of Symeon*, we might say that this person presents us with a hermeneutical choice. Like the fool, they can be dismissed as mad and peripheral, or (and this is perhaps the most common response) as a recipient of care who has nothing further to offer, or as an expression of a form of soft "difference" that invites us into an encounter. Each of these responses, in their own way, end up reinforcing the boundary between the "normal" church and its chaotic "other" and provide us with a way of managing the encounter in a controlled way. The "fool" tradition reminds us, however, that we can make a different choice, to wrestle with the dialectic without being able to foresee or map a path to a harmonious outcome. We can accept the person as a gift, in their radical otherness, prior to raising the question of their value to the community or their role in it. To take this path is to make a theological and ecclesiological decision to treat each member of the community as *placed* there by God even if we may never know why, or how we are to respond.[30]

From the *Life* of Symeon of Emesa, then, we learn something about our earthly church life. What Leontius was witnessing to was the "otherness" of grace, appearing paradoxically on the margins. Like Leontius, we are challenged and changed by unexpected behavior into retelling the story

---

29. Kitwood, *Dementia Reconsidered*, 38–42.
30. Sapp, "Memory."

of the Church differently.³¹ The church is not yet the body of Christ, but is radically incomplete: we can see this from the fact that, often, the fountain of grace has its source outside the church. Paradoxically, this church only starts to *become* the body of Christ when it recognizes its own brokenness, abandons its pretensions to respectability and completeness, opens itself to the wildness of the "other" beyond its walls, and wrestles with the unsolvable mysteries it is presented with. The body of Christ thus discerned is paradoxically related to the visible church and its mundane activity, glimpsed as it loses itself, discerned in patience, metaphor, transgression, and absence.³²

This study of the *Life* of Symeon of Emesa has shed some light on the potential role of people with divergent behavior in the Church. In particular, there are parallels with the positioning of people whose dementia is presenting with unusual and "unmanageable" behaviors that place them outside the prevailing norms of church members. The Church is known as the body of Christ at the point at which it exceeds its self-defined boundaries and surrenders to a dialectical encounter with others who do not and will not fit its expectations. Its members discover their own place within the body at the point at which they recognize their own inability to discern it or establish its norms; they become able to see at the point at which their blindness becomes manifest. The implications of this conclusion will be unpacked in more detail in the next section.

The *Life of Symeon* and the lives of people with dementia in the Church

Although a large proportion of Christian writing on dementia is fairly narrowly focused on fulfilling pastoral needs, there is a richer and deeper current that seeks to establish what dementia and other forms of cognitive impairment may have to say to the Church. The line of thought followed by, for example, Hauerwas in relation to cognitive impairment and most

---

31. "A deepening sense of 'being church' is thus part of the unexpected side of the work of inclusion. . . . Participating in the movement from inclusivity to the spirituality of belonging to one another is an image of the Christian life itself." Saliers, "Spirituality of Inclusiveness," 29.

32. A small but moving example of this process happening in "real time" is the change of heart by Father Kenneth Doyle: see Doyle, "Disruptions."

consistently by Swinton in relation to dementia,[33] portrays the Church as manifesting its essence in the quality of its gentle, inclusive, pastoral care for the most vulnerable. More than that, responding to the most vulnerable gives other Christians the opportunity to practice virtues that are valuable in the whole of their discipleship and to develop habits of patience and openness that are prerequisites for responsiveness to God. Finally, this response helps to realize the Church's mission as it challenges the corrupting narratives in which we are embedded. The Church is the community that enacts the values of the kingdom with the person living with dementia as always already embedded in a network of sanctifying relationships that confer the "identity" thought to have been lost.[34] Thus, for John Swinton, the "malignant social psychology" of Kitwood's account of dementia is an example of one such fallen narrative in a world of corrupt social relations; the redeemed internal relations of the Church should be providing a counter-narrative in which personhood is maintained collectively and "attentiveness" to each other in difference is a key ecclesiological virtue.[35]

There is much more at work here than just pastoral concern of the needy. If, like Symeon, people living with dementia have the capacity to shine a light on our community, then there is the possibility that they will catalyze transformation into closer conformity with the body of Christ, the image of God. Rather than a reduction to sameness, the acceptance of otherness "allows for the road less travelled, allows us to live our life in the way important to us, not necessarily in the way prescribed for us,"[36] and so perhaps be converted. It invites us to a rediscovery of the playfulness and ritual nature of human dialogue.[37] It may drive us to reevaluate the poetic, allusive, and metaphorical ways of interacting that so enrich and undergird Christian worship and that, in our haste and in the excessively literal and linear way in which we expect a conversation to proceed, we have overlooked.[38] It may ultimately lead us to "slow down our thought processes, to become inwardly quiet, to have a kind of poetic awareness; that is, to look

33. Hauerwas, *Suffering Presence*; Swinton, *Becoming Friends of Time*; Swinton, *Dementia*.

34. Linthicum and Hicks, *Redeeming Dementia*; Williams, "Knowing God."

35. Swinton, *Dementia*; Swinton, *Becoming Friends of Time*.

36. Shabahangi, "Redefining Dementia," 4–5.

37. Widdershoven and Berghmans, "Meaning-Making," 187.

38. This is particularly explored in the work of John Killick, who records the words of people with dementia in the form of poetry. See his collection, *You Are Words: Dementia Poems* and, with C. Cordonnier, *Openings: Dementia Poems and Photographs*.

for the significance of metaphor and allusion rather than pursuing meaning with a kind of relentless tunnel vision."[39]

The key strength of this approach is that it is not focused narrowly on the needs of "others," people within or outside the Church, but on the Church's collective and theological nature: what the Church is when the example of Jesus is translated into the life of an historical community. We can see in it a responsiveness to the prophetic challenge to the Church from the "stranger," which has some resemblance to the response of the church of Emesa to Symeon. It recognizes in the challenge presented by those who do not conform to "our" norms the voice of God, converting the church from its enchantment by the secular worldview in which she is immersed and proclaiming the inversion of values that heralds the coming kingdom. The Church welcomes the "stranger" as God's gift even if in doing so it has to abandon its "respectable" values, because the "stranger" brings the call to conversion that makes it the body of Christ.

One of the most detailed and developed outworkings of this principle is in Thomas Reynolds's *Vulnerable Communion*, which arose out of the experience of his son's exclusion from church as a result of a set of complex neurological "disorders" that led to behavioral issues. As well as being an impassioned defense of the principle of inclusion for all in church life, it is a sustained and incisive analysis of the ways in which churches are captured by prevailing ideas of the age in the "cult of normalcy," and what they need to do to realize their true nature as the body of Christ. As I have argued in the case of dementia, so he argues that the "overlooked and often contested 'site'" that is our approach to disability opens up to wider human issues, "bringing to the fore issues of difference, normalcy, embodiment, community, and redemption. For this reason, disability has theological power."[40]

As Symeon's behavior casts a light on the faithlessness and worldliness of the church of his day, so disability and other offenses against "normalcy" expose it for the cult it is: "Human abilities tend to be measured in terms of what is considered normal functioning, wholeness and order, making disability a correlate of dysfunction, incompleteness, and disorder. . . . [I]t is not the impairment itself but the community that is disabling, insofar as it makes rules that draw attention to certain impairments as threats to normal role performances." In its repentance, the community finds its own redemption, since "by way of a critique of normalcy, non-disabled persons

---

39. Tom Kitwood, quoted in Goldsmith, *Hearing the Voice*, 51.
40. Reynolds, *Vulnerable Communion*, 13.

are able to acknowledge their own vulnerability, making possible a broader and richer human solidarity."[41] They are able to see that "all of life comes to us as a gift, an endowment received in countless ways from others throughout our lifetime. When we acknowledge this, the line between giving and receiving, ability and disability, begins to blur."[42]

Thus, to truly *see* and welcome Symeon, or people with disabilities, or those whose behavior has been shaped into unfamiliar forms by dementia, is to be converted. As the community is re-formed along these lines, so it is redeemed, and becomes transformed into the true body of Christ: "Redemption then is a welcoming, an empowering act of divine hospitality. . . . [I]nstead of doing away with impairments and the capacity to suffer, redemption transforms vulnerability into communion with God, prefiguring the final eschatological horizon to come when all things will be so transformed. An entire 'theology of vulnerability' opens up, wherein the marginal and heretofore neglected (i.e. disability) becomes central."[43]

Reynolds's ecclesiology is one in which the mark of the true Church is vulnerability: both of each individual and of the community as a whole as it rejects the safety of the "cult of normalcy" for a society in which the center and the margins are constantly in flux. Its claim to truly be the body of Christ rests on its resemblance to Christ's own life and to the revelation it yields of God's power, "a power that reveals itself through vulnerability. The logic here is paradoxical and subversive. Rather than idealize vulnerability, it produces what I shall call a 'metaphorical reversal' that exposes the false pretenses of the cult of normalcy."[44] With this "metaphorical reversal," the appropriate "positioning" of vulnerable people such as those with disabilities or dementia is not on the periphery of the Church (whence they can be invited in at the discretion of the open-hearted "normal" members) but at the center as Christ's representatives, since radical hospitality is the identifying mark of the Church as body of Christ: "the vulnerable stranger is the one in whom the presence of the divine becomes real. The face of Christ is the face of the stranger."[45]

It would be tempting to settle into this new understanding of the Church, as a place where the stranger becomes a friend or colleague and a

---

41. Reynolds, *Vulnerable Communion*, 15.
42. Reynolds, *Vulnerable Communion*, 14.
43. Reynolds, *Vulnerable Communion*, 19.
44. Reynolds, *Vulnerable Communion*, 19.
45. Reynolds, *Vulnerable Communion*, 245.

"new normal" is established. But, tellingly, Reynold's "vulnerable stranger" is *still* a stranger when they are at the center of the community, and Swinton's "attentiveness to difference" does not erase very profound differences that will continue to challenge and subvert the normative boundaries that the church, as any social and historical institution, must continue to draw and redraw in order to maintain its daily life. Boundaries and expectations cannot be simply abolished, so the life of the Church is at best a sort of permanent revolution in which they are questioned and reshaped.[46]

This brings us to the heart of Reynolds's paradox. It seems we must accept that in reality people who appear to us as "strangers" and "others," including many living with dementia, may find themselves positioned on the edge of the church (albeit, perhaps, as a result of the sin and shortcomings of that church, as Reynolds would point out) and that their role will be expressed in and through that "otherness." But we must at the same time assert that such people are absolutely integral to the Church, since neither they nor their relationship with God have changed in essence and their dementia is part of the journey, not a detour from it. It turns out that the center is the edge, and the edge the center. It turns out that, in its mundane expression, the church only enters into its essence as the body of Christ when it discovers its true center may be outside itself, when it finds itself in its "other."

So the paradox is that the church can only make progress toward its true identity as the body of Christ to the extent that it embraces its "other" and so loses some of its "identity" as a respectably structured and boundaried social institution, over and over again. It starts to become Church as it becomes less recognizably church. There is a parallel here between the ecclesial body of Christ, which manifests its true identity in its own "deconstruction," and the fleshly body of Christ in the previous chapter, which becomes recognizable as the Son of God only as the body is broken down almost to the point of unrecognizability. Because "it is the will of Jesus Christ that the whole body of the Church, no less than the individual members, should resemble Him,"[47] we can retrace in the ecclesial body a parallel process to the redemptive work of Christ in the fleshly body. We will encounter this paradox again in the following chapter on the sacramental

---

46. As Arne Fritzson says in his review of Reynolds's book, just by characterizing people as "disabled" he is already putting them outside the discourse of the "normal": Reynolds does not abolish strangeness and otherness, but seeks to identify the theological significance of it. See Fritzson, Review of *Vulnerable Communion*.

47. Pope Pius XII, *Mystici Corporis*, §47, §54.

body, and I will go on to argue that a similar process is discernible in the journey through dementia itself.

5

"Do you think he has a soul?"
Eucharist, *anamnesis*, and the forgetfulness of dementia

> One tended to speak of him, instinctively, as a spiritual casualty—a "lost soul": was it possible that he had really been "de-souled" by the disease? "Do you think he has a soul?" I once asked the Sisters. They were outraged by my question, but could see why I asked it. "Watch Jimmie in chapel," they said, "and judge for yourself."
>
> I did, and . . . I saw there an intensity and steadiness of attention and concentration that I had never seen before in him or conceived him capable of. I watched him kneel and take the Sacrament on his tongue, and could not doubt the fullness and totality of Communion, the perfect alignment of his spirit with the spirit of the Mass [. . . . He was] absorbed in an act, an act of his whole being, which carried feeling and meaning in an organic continuity and unity.[1]

IN THE PREVIOUS CHAPTER it became clear that there was a paradoxical relationship between the earthly community of Christians and the ecclesial body of Christ that they both are and fail to be. The obvious point at which these two come together is in the sacrament of the eucharist, where (according to Catholic theology) words and actions undertaken by fallible individuals in historical time render the body of Christ present in physical objects, and those participating are also participating in the physical acts of

---

1. Sacks, *Man Who Mistook*, 37.

Jesus at the Last Supper. Equally obviously, if we are seeking an expression of God's presence in the world that is accessible to people regardless of their cognitive or functional capacities, the sacramental grace of the eucharist seems the obvious place to start. It is puzzling, then, that there is very little sacramental theology considering people who live with dementia.[2] Christian writers on Christianity and dementia typically gloss over the sacraments, beyond booklets of practical instruction for how to celebrate them appropriately with those with cognitive impairments.

A case in point, and a good example of why a developed theology of the sacramental body of Christ is necessary and important, can be seen in John Swinton's *Dementia: Living in the Memories of God*.[3] He begins with the questions "Who am I?" and then, "What does it mean to be known, loved and held by God when you have forgotten who God is and you can no longer recognize yourself or those whom you once loved?" and builds an answer throughout the book by an appeal to memory, understood in an expansive way as an active "re-membering." As noted in chapter 2, the theme of God's "re-membering" becomes the basis for an account of the person, of the divine-human relationship, and of the Church as the community of remembering for those who can no longer remember for themselves.

To hold his vision together, Swinton needs a strong and well-articulated theology of the eucharist, in which these three senses of "remembering" unite in a shared divine-human encounter that joins eternity with the present moment in time, in the liturgical meeting of God, individual, and Church. The "hinge" in this argument is between his chapter 8 ("Living in the Memories of God: Memory and Divine Embrace") and chapter 9 ("Becoming Friends of Time: Learning to Live in the Present Moment") when he says,

> Even if our *nephesh* is moving towards its end . . . there are good reasons for hope in the present and for the future. *It is precisely that hope we engage with in the Eucharist.* God's active memory finds embodiment in the community of memory and resurrection. It is here, within that community, that we can discover what God's memory looks like.[4]

But what is extraordinary here is that Swinton does not develop his theology of the eucharist any further. Apart from the occasional mention of

---

2. A notable exception is Schlingheider, "Eucharist, Dementia, and Time."
3. Swinton, *Dementia*.
4. Swinton, *Dementia*, 225–56, my emphasis.

the eucharist in passing, it makes no further appearance in the book (and, significantly, is not mentioned in the index). There is no place here for the action of eucharistic grace.

The purpose of this chapter is to explore the potential of a Catholic theology of the sacraments to resolve this apparent weakness in Swinton's vision and, hopefully, to advance the conversation a little further. In it, I will argue that a developed sacramental theology can on the one hand anchor the notion of a "re-membering God" in a concrete work of divine grace in the messy reality of the everyday; and on the other, locate that act of grace and its recipients in the physical activities that constitute the church community. Within this framework, participation in the sacraments (and particularly in the eucharist) can be understood as the act that truly constitutes us as human persons "before God."

A developed theology of the eucharist along these lines contributes three elements that we can use to understand the story that appears at the beginning of this chapter, the case study of the "Lost Mariner" by the great neurologist Oliver Sacks, and to reflect upon what it may mean for our theology. It enables us to think about Christian faith in ways that are not centered on our ability to understand, remember, or respond over time; it can provide a framework within which we can understand how we are "hidden in the memories of God" by virtue of our membership of the ecclesial body of Christ; and it can reconfigure the concept of memory itself along distinctively Christian and theological lines.

These are large claims, requiring more detailed explanation, analysis, development, and application. The discussion in this chapter will therefore proceed in three stages. First, I shall briefly summarize the current Catholic teaching on the sacraments as presented in the Catechism, and identify the characteristics (its enacted, non-cognitive, non-voluntaristic, collective, physical components) that show most promise for a theology of dementia. I will then explore those elements in more critical and constructive detail in dialogue with three philosophers who build their work out from the twentieth-century phenomenological tradition deriving from the work of Husserl and Heidegger. Finally, I will return to the story with which I began this chapter, the account of the "Lost Mariner," to apply and test the insights gleaned.

Reappraising dementia in the light of Catholic sacramental theology

A convenient starting-point for our exploration of Catholic sacramental theology is the *Catechism of the Catholic Church*, the official summary of Catholic teaching for the instruction of the faithful.[5] Clearly, for the purposes of this study the focus must be on the eucharist as the ecclesial practice that both effects and expresses the communion of Christians in the universal Church,[6] but reference will also be made to baptism as the other universal sacrament and the one in which Christian life and identity originates.

The fundamental principle at work here is that the sacraments are the sovereign work of God, in Christ and through the Holy Spirit (1127). As such they confer the grace they signify *ex opere operato* (literally: "by the very fact of the action's being performed"), i.e., by virtue of the saving work of Christ, accomplished once for all (1128). While the intention, understanding, or disposition of the person receiving this grace may inhibit it from bearing fruit, the initiative and the gift remain God's alone.

The first point of note is that, because of this privileged character, sacramental Christianity obeys a logic of ontological transformation. The elements of the eucharist (the bread and the wine) are transformed into the body and blood of Christ; because of this, those who received them are transformed into the redeemed people of God and sanctified by the Spirit (1364, 1374, 1382). The *anamnesis* (re-calling) of Christ's sacrifice in the elements is reproduced in the recipients; the bread, sanctified through the *epiclesis* (down-calling) of the sanctifying Spirit, is offered to sanctify the people (1129, 1396). The *anamnesis* of Christ's sacrifice and the *epiclesis* of the Spirit are manifested in an act of eternal objectivity that is also specific to a particular community undertaking the sacramental actions in a particular place and time.

There is a circularity here, because the sacraments themselves are celebrated through the work of the people who constitute the Church (*leitourgy*) in union with the eternal heavenly liturgy of Christ (1140). "The liturgy is the work of the whole Christ, head and body. Our high priest celebrates it unceasingly in the heavenly liturgy" (1187). So the fleshly body

---

5. Catholic Church, *Catechism of the Catholic Church*. Numbers in parentheses refer to paragraph numbers in the text.

6. De Lubac, *Corpus Mysticum*.

of Christ is made present as the sacramental body of Christ, which forms and constitutes the ecclesial body of Christ, which in turn in its work represents the sacramental body of Christ.[7] This goes some way further even than Swinton's claim that a person living with dementia who has forgotten him- or herself is nevertheless eternally re-membered by God: where this latter claim is necessarily abstract and dependent on divine sovereignty, the identity constituted by sacramental participation is rooted in an intimate, bodily encounter of person, Church, and God meeting in the eucharistic elements.

The secondary emphasis in this theology lies with human intention, but the stress is no longer on the formation of an individual, conscious intention at a particular point in space and time. It is characteristic of this perspective that intention becomes shared over different time points and different social actors. It is particularly clearly visible in relation to baptism, which is conferred freely on an infant (1250) by virtue of the faith shared through the whole Church. "Faith needs the community of believers. It is only within the faith of the Church that each of the faithful can believe" (1253). But the same principle applies to the eucharist: since the sacraments and the community of the Church are related recursively through the liturgy—the church performs that liturgy that in turn constitutes the church as the body of Christ—the Church "holds" the intention of the individual at times that they are unable to do so. In sacramental theology the concepts of intention and understanding cross time and social space.

Thirdly, "Communion renews, strengthens, and deepens this incorporation into the Church, already achieved by Baptism" (1396). Thus, liturgical and sacramental time takes on a very different character. The eucharist is at once an *anamnesis* of Christ's sacrifice, now present in the liturgy of the Church (1362, 1364) and the eternal banquet of heaven in communion with the resurrected Christ (1382). It is what Kitwood would call a "re-menting" rather than a re-playing,[8] a reversal of our process of forgetting such that the Church "commemorates Christ's Passover, and it is made present: the sacrifice Christ offered once for all on the cross remains ever present" (1364). To participate in one eucharist is thus to participate in *all* eucharists. It follows that the ontological status of the participant "before God" is not dependent on frequency or repetition of the sacraments: to have participated once consciously in the liturgy is to be eternally held

---

7. De Lubac, *Corpus Mysticum*.
8. Kitwood, *Dementia Reconsidered*.

within it and with the community. This is because the eucharist as event is a union with Christ's eternal sacrifice: one may receive the same grace and participate in the same eternal act, although this is manifest in discrete mundane events repeatedly.

At this point it should be possible to discern the outlines of a sacramental theology that addresses the "theological disease" that is dementia. In the face of a progressive loss of memory and executive function, and with the consequent loss of the ability to constitute as a self in time and space, we find that we are constituted in the event of eucharist. *Anamnesis* is not re-playing but re-membering: each celebration of the eucharist is the one original sacrifice and also a unique event in space and time. Each is at once in a chain of continuity stretching back to the Last Supper, and the product of liturgical development and reform affecting every aspect of its performance. If this is a model for "sacred memory," it has implications for how we understand the condition of those who, we believe, are failing to remember events accurately. In the eucharist as in memory, time and eternity meet in a creative act.

This brief survey has brought to light three "convergences" that characterize the event of the eucharist in time and space: between God, individual, and Church all present in an act of copresence; between divine, human, and ecclesiastical intention; and between the present, all pasts, and eternity. Each of these addresses an issue in the theology of dementia: the questions of the person with dementia's "identity" (as located in God and the Church); conscious intent; and status in a time without memory. They provide a framework in which to explore in more detail some current thinking about the eucharist.

Introducing a phenomenological turn

Enlightening as this doctrinal survey is, it does not yet bring new understanding of the human experience of what it is to be a Christian with dementia "before God." For this it is necessary to move the discussion into a different register and explicitly consider receiving the eucharist as an event in the world.[9] The key question will be "What does it mean for human experience to participate in the eucharist (as understood above), and how does this contribute to our theological understanding of living as a Christian with dementia?" To assist us in this task, I will look at three philosophers

9. See Gschwandtner, "Mystery Manifested."

who work within the phenomenological tradition that focuses its attention on the meaning of our experiences as embodied human beings. Each of them attempts an analysis of the eucharist from a different angle, and this triptych of perspectives will contribute to what I hope will be a rounded understanding.

Marion: *The saturated phenomenon and the movement of mutual* kenosis

Jean-Luc Marion has the longest career of the three discussed here, and has been able to develop a fairly comprehensive phenomenological account of the eucharist over the years. His focus is on the eucharist as an event presented to the individual, and its consequences for understanding that individual's standing "before God." Three key moves delineate the outline of his approach.

First, Marion understands the eucharist as the thoroughgoing *kenosis* (emptying-out) of the incarnate God, which in turn has two consequences. One is that, paradoxically, we recognize the self-emptying Christ in the eucharist precisely by the fact that his presence is hidden, that there is no phenomenal sign that the elements are any more than bread and wine, for all signs of divinity have been emptied from the miracle before us. In addition, because Christ is completely incarnated in the bread and wine, our experience of it is a direct experience of God as revealed to us: "To define the phenomenality of the sacrament, one must see that within it the invisible is translated, delivers itself up, and abandons itself to the visible to the point of appearing in it as the invisible that it remains."[10]

But since God cannot be positively experienced in the world in the manner of a created object, God cannot be directly experienced in the eucharist; and this raises the question of what it means to say that the invisible God appears in it as the invisible that God remains. In his second key move, Marion opens the world of divine action to phenomenological analysis via the concept of saturation.[11] In his view, the experience of the eucharist is one of a "divine darkness," an encounter so overwhelming and ineffable that we cannot grasp it or "experience" it at all. He suggests that there is a range of phenomena (such as art, history, culture) that always carry an excess of intuited meanings in a similar way and cannot be reduced to knowledge,

10. Marion, *Believing in Order to See*, 108.
11. Marion, "Saturated Phenomenon."

but are present to us through a "passive synthesis." However, divine revelation is unique in that there is no dimension of its phenomenality that is not saturated:[12] it "saturates phenomenality to the second degree, by saturation of saturation."[13]

Finally, confronted with the dazzling gift of the kenotic Christ in the saturated phenomenon, we know ourselves as *defined* by this gift, as the ones constituted as recipients of the gift: "The sacrament therefore reorients us, makes us devoted or given over to it (*adonné*), as we receive its abandon as far as we are able without exercising control over it, imposing concepts upon it, or determining it in some fashion—all of which would be impossible due to its overwhelming character."[14] The only appropriate and wholly complete response is one of kenotic abandon: we are no longer responsible for constituting our own identities as individual cognitive subjects.

In Marion's account of the eucharist, there is an objectivity and intensity of focus at the point of reception: we are required to bring no memory, intentionality, self-insight, or knowledge to this eternal moment; our response is of a responding kenotic abandonment. We are required only to receive the Christ who has abandoned his own identity to the moment with an answering self-abandon, to give over our own selves to the moment of communion with the body of Christ. It is in this way that we are constituted as subjects before God. For Marion, therefore, the deficits represented by dementia have no necessary relevance, because we are not in the world of knowledge or understanding.

Falque: The eucharist as mediated body-to-body

Emmanuel Falque can be understood to add to Marion's "saturated event" a phenomenological analysis of the human response. He brings to the question a concern to recover the lost bodiliness of the encounter in the eucharist, because "when we talk [in phenomenology] of the 'flesh' we describe the *lived experience* of our bodies . . . while we also bracket off the *organic quality* of the 'body.' . . . Our difficulty in that respect makes it almost impossible to think seriously about the organic at the heart of the Resurrection."[15] This is a mistake, because it is in our organic nature

12. Marion, *Being Given*, 235.
13. MacKinlay, "Eyes Wide Shut," 448.
14. Gschwandtner, "Mystery Manifested," 319.
15. Falque, *Wedding Feast*, 1–2.

that we become most keenly aware of the abyss of emptiness upon which humankind is constructed, and where that abyss is ultimately overcome by the resurrection of Christ. For Falque, human existence teeters on the edge of primeval chaos, the *tōhû-wābōhû* of Genesis 1, from which we are created and to which we are destined to return. Our salvation comes *through* the chaos in the form of the resurrected Christ, who is present to us in the sacrament. We receive the benefit of this salvation not primarily through an act of intention, remembrance, or cognitive ability, but through the very physical act of chewing ("manducation") the piece of bread that has become the physical body of Christ.

Falque's argument is a wide-ranging and complex one and no attempt will be made to summarize it in its entirety here, but it culminates in an intensive focus on the phenomenology of the reception of the eucharist as an act of physical manducation and digestion. He seeks to "try to think through the transformation of our embodiedness in the act of the eucharist (eucharistic *content*), having rooted it in an animality that is converted into humanity by recognition of its filiation (eucharistic *heritage*) and before performing the donation in an agape that loses nothing of its erotic genesis even in relinquishing its own body to the body of the other (eucharistic *modality*)."[16]

This approach has distinct contributions to make to the discussion here. The first is that, in Falque's description of the abyss, there are strong resemblances to the descriptions of dementia that underlie its power and importance as a "theological disease" but also a proposed solution: "we become formless there. We break up. We are first of all ruined there, spoiled, like objects that fall and collide. But then there is more and better in the abyss, which takes the place and role of finitude, once there is a question of the eucharist . . . ."[17] There is something of an echo here of Marion's process of mutual *kenosis* in the reception of the eucharist: as our personhood dissolves into the chaos of the abyss, so we encounter in the eucharistic elements the Christ who emptied himself and gave himself up even to our manducation and digestion!

The next contribution is that, because of his organic approach to the union of Christ and the recipient in the eucharist, Falque can take leave of an approach to the sacrament exclusively through consciousness and conscious memory. Memory is a whole-body phenomenon that will not be

16. Falque, *Wedding Feast*, 199.
17. Falque, *Wedding Feast*, 6.

reduced to consciousness, and remembrance is a physical act rather than a passive recall of past events. "Because we participate in the Mass consciously, or rather, through our consciousness, we are inclined to forget the silent experience of the body-to-body [*corps à corps*] of human and God .... The memory is inscribed, or should be inscribed, in our own bodies—just as the memory of food leads us always, almost biologically, to look for it."[18] He concludes that "the memory of the Last Supper is, then, a memory of the body, and not simply an epiphenomenon of the consciousness piled upon the brain."[19]

This opens a way of thinking about the relationship between God and the person with dementia, and of the sacramental event as "inscribed in our bodies" regardless of whether we have a conscious memory of it, that is reminiscent of Swinton's discussion of memory as a "whole-body" phenomenon.[20] Gabrielli comments, "Taking up the liturgical anamnesis, Falque points out what scientists continue to uncover: that memory is not merely a conceptual faculty. If it were, one might suppose a simple recollection of Christ could be enough. But we're embodied. . . . Thus, the Eucharist draws to light the fundamental bodiliness of memory. We remember in, through, and by our bodies. God's becoming body makes clear that 'actually, the whole body must participate' in the sacrifice made for us."[21] This insight will become particularly important when, in chapter 7, we turn to consider my mother's last day: when, in late-stage dementia, her body appears to be the only medium through which she can respond to the call of her God.

Finally (and perhaps most strikingly), Falque sees the act of our reception of Christ in the sacrament as one half of a double movement, in which we are incorporated into Christ's body even as we incorporate (through eating) his body into ours. The communion "is not satisfying simply because of the presence of a small Jesus at its heart. . . . Nobody simply eats God, but we are always in some respect eaten by him. From our being anthropophagous (eating the body of Christ) what becomes clear is a kind of theophagy (to be eaten or incorporated into the body of Christ)."[22] Thus, on the one hand "it is a life of God that weaves its way like the ineffable

---

18. Falque, *Wedding Feast*, 210–11.
19. Falque, *Wedding Feast*, 212.
20. Swinton, *Dementia*.
21. Gabrielli, Review of *The Wedding Feast of the Lamb*.
22. Falque, *Wedding Feast*, 205.

and discreet movement of blood in our vascular system," and on the other, "that which is assimilated by us, in the unique case of the body of Christ, is what assimilates us; or rather, paradoxically, it incorporates us even into Christ-there whom we eat."[23] This almost completely erases the distinction between Christ's fleshly body and the Church as body of Christ: we (collectively) become part of Christ's flesh at the moment that he becomes part of ours as individuals. For the same reason, the distinction between each of us is erased as we become, literally, one flesh. "Finally we arrive at 'the flesh in common' as embodiedness shared and, at last, achieved in part. With the eucharistic viaticum there is a community of embodiedness for us today, *in via*, and not just the satisfaction of our individualities hereafter, *in patria*."[24]

Gschwandtner: The phenomenology of this particular event

Christina Gschwandtner is a scholar of modern French thinkers of theology in a phenomenological mode, and her work has strongly influenced the whole of this chapter. In a critical survey of the work of Marion, Falque, and Lacoste she criticizes Marion and Falque as "still too prone to consider the eucharist in isolation from its liturgical and ritual context. For this reason, these analyses of the phenomenality of the eucharist tend to describe it as a solitary and excessive phenomenon, disregarding the corporate, corporeal, and communal dimensions of eucharistic experience within its liturgical setting."[25] This setting, she says, is also part of the phenomenological analysis of the eucharist, since the context cannot be separated from the rite itself:

> Eucharist is also always experienced at a specific time and place [which] function to situate the experience of the eucharist. . . . [I]t is never a disembodied, atemporal, aspatial experience, but always one that involves setting aside time, coming into a place, as well as corporeal movement and gesture. This corporeal dimension is immensely important: participants bow or kneel, fold their hands or open them for reception, come forward, cross themselves or fold their hands over their chest, kneel at an altar rail, and ultimately return to their seats or place to stand, finally leaving the church

---

23. Falque, *Wedding Feast*, 206.
24. Falque, *Wedding Feast*, 231.
25. Gschwandtner, "Mystery Manifested," 316.

altogether, yet maybe with the taste of wine and bread still on their lips.[26]

Within this specific time and place, memory, intention, and conscious awareness are interwoven into a complex fabric of circumstance and experience. In the moment of the event itself there is a layering of memory and anticipation: of past and future eucharists, and of the succession of events comprising the present eucharistic celebration. "The 'moment' of eucharistic participation is thus distended through memory and anticipation."[27]

Discernible behind this "extended moment" of participation is a rich and complex backdrop that provides its context and frame. In the first place, it must be viewed against a "larger liturgical horizon: as part of an extended ceremony that itself is part of a liturgical week and year, a larger liturgical temporality that gives meaning to the particular experience."[28] Secondly, there is a web of affective cues: entry to the "sacred" building, smells, sounds, tastes, movements, as well as sights that are collectively reinforced by the repetitive and recursive character of this liturgy and the liturgical cycle. Finally, and because of this communal liturgical horizon, the liturgy shapes intentionality in a distinctive way that is not ultimately dependent upon a conscious choice:

> Regular participants in liturgy become habituated to it; its modes of repetition function to inscribe it on their bodies, generating consistent emotions or moods of expectation. In this way, the larger liturgical context forms a liturgical disposition that is marked in sensorial, affective, and corporeal ways. Our bodies and emotions become prepared for liturgy and eucharist through the cycles of repetition and the habituation they engender. . . . The liturgy forms a disposition and expectation, that is, an intentionality that prepares consciousness to intend and receive eucharist in particular ways.[29]

Thus, and in distinction to both Marion and Falque, Gschwandtner draws out the essentially communal character of the eucharist, which through all these ways "shapes an experience that at least for a short time knits us together as one."[30] It is therefore the activity of the community that

---

26. Gschwandtner, "Mystery Manifested," 326.
27. Gschwandtner, "Mystery Manifested," 326.
28. Gschwandtner, "Mystery Manifested," 327.
29. Gschwandtner, "Mystery Manifested," 328.
30. Gschwandtner, "Mystery Manifested," 328.

shapes the intentional behavior of the recipient of the eucharist, rather than *vice versa*. We come to the eucharist not with our intention fully formed, but as potential participants, open to the capacity of elements of the liturgy (and our shared sedimented memory of previous instances) to shape us into a community that is, collectively, consciously and intentionally open to sacramental grace.

Gschwandtner's contribution brings the discussion of the eucharist back "down to earth," rooting it in the historical practices of the worshiping community, and completes the triptych of perspectives I have summarized for the sake of this argument. Although she makes more use of the concepts of memory and intentionality than either of the previous two contributors, she embeds both in the web of meanings, practices, associations, and repetitive behaviors of the historical community: neither memory nor intentionality are the products of the individual consciousness of the subject, but can be understood as held collectively and communally.

To summarize, we have arrived at a rich description of the eucharist that addresses the three critical issues of the participant's identity, intentionality, and memory. For Marion, the regulative idea is the "saturated experience" of God's epiphany in the eucharist, beyond conscious cognition or personal "re-collection," a kenotic gift beyond grasping or placing in a temporal sequence, that draws from us an answering act of self-emptying that constitutes us "before God." For Falque, the constituting divine–human encounter is as one body to another, a connection of manducation and mutual absorption more profound and organic than conscious intention or memory. For Gschwandtner this encounter is not separable from the liturgical life of the Church, which stages the *anamnesis* of the divine–human encounter in a web of reiterated and elaborated words, practices, and symbols that situate the participants and collectively form their intention without, necessarily, conscious activity on their part. It now remains to test this broad picture by applying it to a particular case, in order to see whether it has some capacity to cast additional light on the issues it raises. For this, I will return to the story with which this chapter begins.

Rescuing the Lost Mariner

Oliver Sacks was an eminent neurologist whose literary output largely comprised reflections on case studies of individuals with particular neurological disorders. "The Lost Mariner" is perhaps his most famous and presents the case of Jimmie G, a former sailor who was perpetually marooned by his dementia (Korsakoff syndrome)[31] in the late 1940s. Jimmie's inability to form new memories meant that he was unable to focus and seemed incapable of feeling deeply or empathizing for long with those around him. It is his story that heads this chapter.

For Sacks himself, this incident speaks of the power of feeling—of the aesthetic and emotional—to integrate Jimmie's scattered personhood, rendering him for a while "deeply attentive to the beauty and soul of the world."[32] Sacks's interpretation reflects his presuppositions as a secular, rationalist clinician. Swinton interprets the story from a more theologically and pastorally informed perspective, and presents us with the possibility that, at times like this, there is more going on theologically than a mere conditioned response to familiar stimuli:

> when a person is caught up in a familiar prayer or hymn, or when they simply clap their hands to the rhythm of a song, they may well be remembering, cognitively or bodily, experiences they have had with God—or they may be having an experience with God at that very moment.... We do people who suffer from dementia a huge disservice if we simply assume that their moments of "springing to life" are nothing but instances of meaningless procedural memory.[33]

This is profound and important as far as it goes, but also reflects Swinton's theological starting-point in the assumption that the eucharist is one of a range of doxological options that all express, but cannot be said to constitute, the identity of the Christian "before God." In this chapter I have started from a different set of assumptions that takes the sacraments as foundational. Taking that as our interpretative starting-point, how else may this story be read?

Taking our cue from Marion, we may say that we are witnessing here the phenomenology of Jimmie's encounter with God-as-saturated-phenomenon. The majority of the time, this encounter is veiled in the perfect *kenosis* of the incarnate God, to the point that, intellectually, we can identify nothing in the sacrament that is not of the attributes of bread and wine. Perhaps, freed from this need to attempt to cognitively grasp the saturated

---

31. See https://www.alz.org/alzheimers-dementia/what-is-dementia/types-of-dementia/korsakoff-syndrome for a summary of the main features of this syndrome.

32. Sacks, *Man Who Mistook*, 37.

33. Swinton, *Dementia*, 251.

event, we see in Jimmie one who is constituted and knows himself as the *adonné* and gives himself wholly over to it. When the "Lost Mariner" loses himself in God, he is found again.

Following Falque, we may focus on the moment when Jimmie receives the sacrament on his tongue as "the perfect alignment of his spirit with the spirit of the Mass." By encountering Christ body-to-body, in the knowledge of his whole organic body, he comes to a "knowledge" that transcends cognition or memory. As Jimmie digests the body of Christ and it enters into his inner chaos, so he is "digested" into eternal membership in the same body of Christ, finds his resurrection and inner coherence as participator in the ordered kingdom of God. By meeting Christ in the chaos of the abyss, he is brought back to life.

Turning, finally, to Gschwandtner, we might note the circumstances of this moment of transformation in the space and time of the Church: the eternal series of repetitions stretching back, not just to the 1940s but to the Last Supper itself, within which this Mass is located as a moment in a liturgical journey; the collective memory and intentionality that re-members and prepares for this sacramental moment; and the rich abundance of sensory cues that shape, prepare, and orient Jimmie's consciousness irrespective of his capacity to direct his own attention to that moment.

This brings us back to Swinton's discussion, with a consideration of how the (liturgical and pastoral) practices of the church community support and enrich the eucharistic process. For Swinton these practices include attending to the present moment, along with naming and holding the person; with Gschwandtner, we may further see these practices as an expression of the eucharistic grace in which we are each bedazzled by the divine gift, drawn into the body of Christ and so shaped to our very core by its practices and presence.

Swinton began his book with Bonhoeffer's specific question, "Who am I?" and the more pointed supplementary, "What does it mean to be known, loved and held by God when you have forgotten who God is and you can no longer recognize yourself or those whom you once loved?"[34] In his response, he presents a palette of meditations and reflections that provide a rich answer but do not develop the sacramental dimension in much detail. In this chapter, I have explored what eucharistic theology might have to add to our emerging Christian understanding of dementia. Clearly, the world of sacramental theology is extensive and elaborate, and there is much

---

34. Swinton, *Dementia*, 4–5.

more that may emerge as the territory is explored further. However, two points have emerged in this discussion that need to be taken forward in later chapters.

First, there is a clearer sense of the ways in which the accounts of the body of Christ in this and the two previous chapters fit together: notwithstanding the subtitle of this book, we are not talking of three different "bodies," but three senses in which we encounter the Christ who knows and completes us. Thus, what we encounter in the eucharist is the Christ who shares in the same physicality as ourselves in the life of Jesus, and the same "deconstruction incarnate" on the cross: "In pouring the divine self into the world, God affirms the embodied creature. Such an incarnational vision radiates sacramental power. Not only is humanity created in God's image; God also draws near to abide in, validate and empower human vulnerability as loved by God."[35]

Equally, in the eucharist we encounter and become once again members of the ecclesial body of Christ who offer the sacrifice of his body in his name: "Wholeness is joyfully celebrated at the Eucharistic meal where we actually become, again and again, members of one body.... When the Spirit aids our remembrance, we are truly remembered. This signifies profound hope for those who are *de-mented*; who now in Christ become *re-mented*, *re-minded*, *re-membered*. The tragedy for the church is that those who can remember, too often forget to remember to include in worship, those who have forgotten that they cannot remember."[36]

Secondly, there is a distinct pattern emerging here, regarding how we encounter and recognize the body of Christ in these distinct instantiations. In chapter 3, we found that it is at the point that Christ "loses his identity" as a distinct physical body with clear boundaries and a cognitively composed centre that he is manifest as the Son of God. In the next chapter, I argued that the mundane church only shows itself to be the ecclesial body of Christ at the point at which it abandons its sense of identity, recognizes that it is *not* fulfilling that vocation, and stands in need of intervention from the margins. In this chapter, it is as Christ becomes undetectable under the form of the bread and the wine (except to the eyes of faith) that he becomes knowable by Jimmie: Christ's loss of a discreet identity becomes, paradoxically, the place in which he is most himself in the body of Christ, and under that form he meets Jimmie in the abyss of forgetfulness.

---

35. Reynolds, *Vulnerable Communion*, 202.
36. Hudson, "God's Faithfulness," 61.

These findings have implications for how we understand ourselves and our discipleship, with dementia or without. Called into communion with and as the body of Christ, we find ourselves constituted and sanctified by it; in our fallible bodies and minds, and through their fallibility in solidarity with his. Called into conformity with the same Christ, the perfect Image of God, we find a persistent theme running through it: that Christ's body is recognizable in its full glory only when it loses its "identity," when it becomes reduced to broken fragments of flesh, an unbounded collectivity, or a piece of food to be chewed. It seems we know Christ's body by its *ungraspability*, by the ways in which it cannot be defined, analyzed, or identified as a commodity in our world. By extension, it may be that we become fully ourselves in Christ when we too become ungraspable, when we do not have the familiar markers of an "identity" in the eyes of others and are knowable more truly through our different participations in the body of Christ. The insights from this chapter have implications for how we understand the Christian journey of faith and discipleship—through the successive stages of dementia and ultimately as fulfilled in the eschatological kingdom—which I will be exploring in the next one.

6

From cognition, through emotion, into spirit

Continuing faith in the midst of dementia

As my mother's dementia progressed, her faith remained firm even as her grasp of its content and forms slipped away. There was a period in which, whenever we met, she would insist that we prayed. We would put our hands together and bow our heads, and she would adopt a "prayerful" voice as she led us in devotions that did not "make sense" in sentences or even complete words. But they made sense to her, it seems.

Mum, a fairly traditional Baptist, would have been impatient of "vain repetition" or "empty babbling" in prayer, and stressed the importance of individual, intentional faith. As her son, I was left with some questions. Can we say that there was an intention there beyond the words, that the Spirit's intercession "with groans too deep for words" was enough? When the world is no longer constructed in concepts and sentences, what happens to prayer? And what happens to my mother's decades-old faith?

So far, I have suggested that we start with our humanity in the image of God (understood as our acceptance of the life given to us by God) and growing into God's likeness (understood as the likeness of Christ). I went on to argue that the context for this is Christ's solidarity with and presence to us in the "three bodies of Christ" which provide the context, grace, and exemplar for our journey. We must now turn to the question of what it might mean to grow into the "image and likeness" of God in the midst of dementia.

If, as I am proposing, God draws close and shares in the life of the person living with dementia, then we can learn something important about this God and our vocation in God's image and likeness by paying close attention to their faith journey. We can learn something important about faith in general by paying attention to how a person of faith who lives with dementia grows and changes along the way, an insight that acts as a potential counterweight to the Church's emphasis on holding particular thoughts, engaging in particular practices, or carrying out particular actions. We may learn what faith would look like, delivered from our idolatrous attachment to hypercognitivity and performative competence. We may also learn what we can hope for and aspire to, if our own journey toward union with God takes us through the vale of dementia.

Two assumptions underlie this chapter. The first is that faith itself cannot be compromised or impaired merely by the impairments of dementia. The second is that the shape, depth, and expression of that faith will necessarily change and progress as the dementia progresses. An individual's faith is always changing as their circumstances change, as new challenges arise bringing new opportunities for growth. The challenge for us is to identify the continuing work of the Spirit in the faith of the individual-in-communion even as somebody's capacity to conceptualize and communicate in conventional sentences deteriorates and the traditional expressions of the faith in word and gesture become less and less obvious.

These assumptions rule out what I have elsewhere referred to as the "palliative" approach to the spirituality and faith-journey of Christians with dementia: the assumption that in this case there are no challenges to be met, mountains to climb, or depths of encounter with God to be plumbed, but only the need to be "kept comfortable" with familiar religious tropes, reassurance, and the religious equivalent of pain relief.[1] On the contrary, they mean we must take it as given that such a person continues as a Christian disciple and even a sort of "spiritual pioneer."

Speaking of the process of growing old, Pope Francis points out that "this period of life is different from those before, there is no doubt; we even have to somewhat 'invent it ourselves,' because our societies are not ready, spiritually and morally, to appreciate the true value of this stage of life.

---

1. Kevern, "Spirituality and Dementia."

Indeed, it once was not so normal to have time available; it is much more so today. Christian spirituality has also been caught somewhat by surprise, with regard to outlining a kind of spirituality of the elderly."[2] If this is true of old age in general, it is perhaps true of the experience of dementia in particular. In terms of Christian spirituality, we have been "caught by surprise" by dementia; and if we wish to understand how the relationship with God through Christ changes as dementia progresses, the people we need to consult are those who have experienced it. The focus of this chapter will therefore be on what they can show us as they "invent it themselves," either in their own words or by a careful process of social reconstruction.

From cognition, through emotion, into spirit

It is undoubtedly the case that every person's faith-journey through dementia is different, so generalizations must be made with some care. But Christine Bryden's reflection on her own faith-journey may provide us with a starting-point:

> I believe that people with dementia are making an important journey from cognition, through emotion, into spirit. I've begun to realize what really remains throughout this journey is what is really important, and what disappears is what is not important. I think that if society could appreciate this, then people with dementia would be respected and treasured.[3]

This account of a journey "from cognition, through emotion, into spirit" has an authority and persuasiveness for several reasons. In the first place, it echoes a long tradition of Catholic mysticism that sees our journey to God in three stages: purgation (when the emphasis is on the cultivation of virtue through intentional activity); illumination (characterized both by joy in the felt presence of God and desolation in God's perceived absence) and union (characterized by self-forgetfulness and abstraction from earthly things).[4] Secondly, it seems to capture some of the clinical features typical of cognitive loss in many cases of dementia: first the explicit, discursive capacity starts to erode, exposing the longer-lasting emotional life in its intensity; then, as this deteriorates, what is left is a sort of stillness as language

---

2. Pope Francis, "General Audience."
3. Bryden, *Dancing*, 159.
4. Garrigou-Lagrange, *Three Ages*.

is lost and a silence persists, punctuated only by the more or less habitual actions of "muscle memory"—a process that David Vance memorably likened to the way in which an encroaching tide first exposes, then washes away each successive stratum on the beach.[5] Finally, it reflects a very practical distinction that is widely made between early-, middle-, and late-stage dementia, where the early stage is characterized by initial difficulties with activities of daily living, the middle stage by increasing need for care and support from others, and the late stage by loss of ability to communicate, disengagement from surroundings, and difficulty with basic skills such as eating and swallowing.

This alignment of different three-stage schemes may seem whimsical, but I believe it shows us something important, in the way it links together a progress in the faith with a loss of cognitive and performative capacity, and allows us to make connections between these very different worlds. It also draws attention to the likely fact that, at each of those stages, the spirituality of the person concerned will undergo significant changes. It will not only change in term of its challenges (such as loss of independence) and the ways in which it is resourced and expressed (such as through beliefs, rituals, or songs) but in the very definition of "spirituality" that we use. Will we focus on peoples' statements about their belief, or their expressions of emotion? When even emotion seems beyond the reach of understanding or interpretation, what will we count as "spirituality"? While it is possible to overdraw the distinction between each of the three stages in the progress of dementia—every individual is different, and in none of them is the transition from one stage to another clearly marked—it seems natural and appropriate to talk of three approaches to "spirituality" corresponding to these three notional stages. Of these, it is the last two stages that deserve the most attention, and I will devote a chapter to each one.

I do not intend to spend much time considering how faith changes and grows in the early stage of dementia, when it is interfering with the person's life but has not yet undermined their capacity to think and respond in their accustomed ways. At this stage, faith can still adapt within a discursive frame: for example, MacKinlay and Trevitt in their study of the spirituality of people with early-stage dementia found that the faith challenges and insights were comparable to others of the same age without dementia.[6] The resources of faith developed over the course of a life prior to the onset of

---

5. Vance et al., "Practical Implications," 24.
6. Trevitt and MacKinlay, "'Just Because.'"

dementia—religious practices, discourse, social networks—are still largely available to the disciple at this stage of the dementia journey and so the challenge is to shape the faith story so as to take account of dementia and its challenges. The experience of dementia in this stage is typically one of loss, vulnerability, and disconnection both from others and from oneself, and the disciple with dementia may respond proactively to address these feelings; but they can do so with the full range of their accustomed spiritual tools.[7]

In short, the majority of what we have from people who are living with dementia at this stage could be broadly termed "religious coping," adaptations to one's faith in response to the new challenge.[8] Thus, for example, Patricia Williams's study of evangelicals with a diagnosis of dementia in "early to moderate stages" catalogues five main ways in which the participants in her study juxtaposed their reflections on their faith with their experience of dementia, all unequivocally affirmative of God's continuing care and their continuing faith.[9] Jennifer Bute found her faith was sufficiently well-founded that dementia presented her with a "glorious opportunity" to extend her ministry by explaining the experience of dementia and developing new treatments "as an insider," while supported by the miraculous intervention of miracles and angels when in danger.[10] Tamara Horsburgh's work with Christians who had a diagnosis of dementia, mostly in the early stage, found them actively reflecting theologically and maintaining their faith in the face of adversity.[11] Inspiring as these stories are, they do not challenge the way we understand faith itself, and need not detain us for long here. It seems the spiritual work of early-stage dementia is of acceptance and reframing, finding the same God in the face of fear and change. The main body of this chapter, therefore, will consider how that spirituality may change as the person's ability to deploy their favored tools in the service of religious coping is impaired.

---

7. Beuscher and Grando, "Using Spirituality"; Beuscher and Beck, "Literature Review."
8. Emery and Pargament, "Religious Coping."
9. Williams, *God's Not Forgotten Me*.
10. Bute and Morse, *Dementia from the Inside*.
11. Horsburgh, *Impact of Holding Faith*.

From cognition, through emotion, into spirit

When prayers stop making sense

Things start to change profoundly as a person who has dementia enters the middle stage of the condition when, as Bryden puts it, they start to move "from cognition, through emotion." The changes that, collectively, are grouped into the broad category of mid-stage dementia are ones that reduce the capacity for a spirituality based upon thinking: they make it harder to create a coherent self-narrative and to frame faith in God in abstract and systematic ways. From a conventional theological point of view, they may be understood to generate a "transcendence deficit" as the capacity to engage with deep questions of meaning is impaired.[12] So, for example, Cook discusses whether we can consider dementia as a "malaise of immanence": "The person who suffers from one of the dementias might often be understood as imprisoned within an immanent frame of reference . . . . [T]he capacity for complex, 'transcendent' and self-reflective thought is impaired and—eventually—largely lost. . . . Everyday life becomes flat and ordinary at best, frightening and overwhelming at worst."[13]

If this were the only spiritual change taking place in the progression of dementia, we may well be justified in understanding it straightforwardly as a loss of spiritual capacity. However, the "transcendence deficit" referred to in the previous paragraph is not a loss of ability to *respond* to the transcendent God, but a loss of the capacity to *conceptualize* God in abstract terms. As the regulatory role of the intellect is impaired, there is the possibility of an intuitive relationship to God that is more vivid, not less. This progression, from a transcendently oriented faith to one more intimate, intuitive, and personal, is reproduced in the account of Robert Davis. A US Baptist pastor, he felt that many of the supports he had grown used to in his faith were slipping away from him. There is for him no "sixth sense" that feels God's presence. Instead, he contemplates the future as one of loss of faith, and the distant hope of its resurrection after death:

> Now I discovered the cruelest blow of all. This personal, tender relationship that I had with the Lord was no longer there. This time of love and worship was removed. There were no longer any feelings of peace and joy. I cried out to God for it to be restored. I howled out to the Lord to come back and speak to my spirit as he had done before. . . . "O God, I have lost so much already! How can

12. Collicutt, "Spiritual Awareness," 22.
13. Cook, "Lived Experience," 92.

you take this last joy from me? Why have you made my sunlight turn into moonlight?"[14]

However, in this case, Davis finds spiritual consolation returning to him via a different, less cognitively oriented route:

> The sweet, holy presence of Christ came to me. He spoke to my spirit and said, "Take my Peace. Stop your struggling. This is all in keeping with my will for your life . . . ." In my confused and shattered emotional condition, Christ had to meet me in this special way. He adjusted his way of comforting me so that it would immerse me in the radiance of his very presence.[15]

With the progression of dementia, the character of faith is changing (as Bryden would put it, "from cognition to emotion"): new characteristics are coming to the fore and the emotional, affective content of the faith is taking on a less mediated role. So, for example, Snyder recounts the story of "a Catholic man" who found that, paradoxically, the loss of some aspects of his religion left him with more faith:

> I no longer remember prayers I once recited automatically. The prayers frequently get mixed up with each other. . . . As for the sacrament of penance or confession it too requires memory. I do not recall when I last went to confession or how many sins I have committed or what in fact sin is, especially if it is non-physical. I don't know if I know all manner of right and wrong—it is more of a feeling of what is right and wrong. . . . I am less Catholic now. I didn't mean or want it to happen; it just did. However, God is in my heart. Somehow he connects to me physically. I think this feeling is called spirituality. There is a sixth sense at work that feels his presence. I talk to God because I do not remember prayer. . . . I don't understand how one could become less religious and possibly more spiritual. Yet this appears to be happening.[16]

While it is clear from these accounts that people encounter God throughout their journey through the middle stages of dementia, it may still seem that this is a reduced and individualist encounter, a consolation for the loss of transcendence, loss of openness to past and future, the lack of a future as a "spiritual pioneer." However, there is no simple connection between the loss of conceptual capacity and the loss of all transcendence from

14. Davis and Davis, *My Journey*, 47.
15. Davis and Davis, *My Journey*, 54–55.
16. Snyder, "Satisfactions and Challenges," 311.

the life of a person with mid-stage dementia, and Cook's diagnosis of dementia as a "malaise of immanence" should not be understood in absolute terms. As he himself points out, to be human is to live between immanence and transcendence in dynamic relationship, and were we to lose one pole entirely, we would not be fully human. It must be the case therefore that "when we are most reduced to the limits of immanent experience, there we find ourselves no less close to transcendent encounter. Thus, within each present moment of the lived experience of dementia, the possibility of a transcendent encounter remains."[17] Although this opening-out to the infinite may not be manageable in cognitive terms, the same limitations that opened the hearts of some of the people in this chapter to immanence may also be releasing them into a different sort of transcendence, and this will repay closer attention.

Return to transcendence

At the same time as cognitive, language, and communication skills may be becoming eroded, meaning-making may be growing less regulated. For Naomi Feil, founder of "Validation Therapy," this is an inevitable developmental stage: discursive language becomes less important while objects and gestures remain freighted with symbolic meaning; conscious memory is replaced by links between events that elicit emotions in the present and those eliciting the same emotions in the past; inner intuition takes on increased salience as the external senses, or the ability to interpret their input accurately, fade.[18] Personhood is changing, and with it the landscape of the faith. What does faith look like, what are its challenges and insights, in this new landscape of dementia?

The key to understanding what may be going on lies with the concept of metaphor, when the uncontrollable play of meanings across words and verbal images opens us up to unimagined vistas, sensitizes us to intuitions that seem too big for us to manage. This is the sort of understanding of metaphor developed by Paul Ricoeur, who argues that putting together two incompatible ideas or images in a sentence creates a sort of shock that forces us to look for the resemblance; and that in this activity, brand new meanings emerge.[19] Metaphor allows us to gesture toward something, reach for

17. Cook, "Lived Experience," 96.
18. De Klerk-Rubin and Potts, "Validation Method."
19. Ricoeur, *Interpretation Theory*, 52–53. See also Harkaway-Krieger, "Theology and Theories of Metaphor."

it without grasping: it is, perhaps, "the only possible language available to religion because it alone is honest about Mystery."[20]

Is it possible, then, that some people entering the middle stages of dementia find themselves opening to mystery as their language and worldview become more metaphorical? John Killick, a poet who works with people who live with dementia, paying careful attention to their words and turning them into expressive poetry, indicates that they may:

> A significant characteristic of the speech of many people with dementia is the direct expression of emotion. The disease has a disinhibiting effect and so the barrier to speaking directly of one's feelings has been swept away. At the same time intellectual capacities are diminished, and rational language proves elusive. Suddenly talk blooms with metaphor, allusion, the currents of feeling are reflected in rhythm and cadence. I have no doubt that the natural language of those with dementia is poetry.[21]

In a later work, he points to the extraordinary vividness that peoples' words can have when detached from too-precise structures of meaning[22] and goes on to quote Karen Hayes:

> People with dementia very often seem to see more than we do, to see through things, round things, past things. Their senses appear at times to be differently deployed so that they hear smells, see voices, taste pictures. They use metaphor as we might use observation, their linguistic range which to us without dementia may appear very strangely configured, is also fluid, generously, even lavishly, overlaid with imagery, freed from grammatical or chronological rules. It is already poetic in essence.[23]

Killick tries to preserve this freshness and directness in the poetry that he crafts from the words spoken to him over the course of a day or even longer. Most of the poems that Killick crafts from the speech of his interlocutors with dementia are not explicitly "spiritual," of course: rather, the wonder of life, its beguiling mystery, shine through the gaps that open up in mundane conversations, lists of objects, fragmentary stories. Occasionally, however, the spiritual wisdom makes itself heard in a more direct way:

---

20. Rohr, *Immortal Diamond*, 58.
21. Killick, *You Are Words*, 7.
22. Killick, *Poetry and Dementia*, 11.
23. Hayes, "Landscape of Dementia."

Glimpses

to see what is beautiful
to hear what is beautiful
they don't know what is beautiful

all these young people
good men, nice boys, fine chaps—
they are too busy to see

it'll be a good bit longer
before you see
what you want to see

but they don't want to see
what in some queer way
they are anxious to see

we see it very rarely
but the difference is
we are trying to see![24]

Perhaps, then, the loss of some cognitive and linguistic capacities need not lead to a diminishment of somebody's spirituality, a narrowing of the breadth of their relationship with God. Perhaps it can lead to a new directness, a new openness and creativity as, in dementia, we are freed to use what remains of language in ways that open us more directly to experience, to an encounter with God untrammeled by old formulae and "dead metaphors." Perhaps the need to find new ways to express accustomed truths opens us to strange new associations and vivid new imagery, for "the creation or discovery of a living metaphor is part of how a human being puts language to their experience, part of how we understand and communicate something new."[25]

Similarly, the practice of worship and adoration may remain in all its richness while perhaps becoming disinhibited. We encountered this phenomenon earlier in the story of the "Lost Mariner," and arguably also in the behavior of Symeon the holy fool. As is widely attested, the symbolic richness and habituated practice of worship may elicit an emotional world that remains alive and inviting for a person of faith with dementia. For example, MacKinlay recounts the case of a woman with advanced dementia who "still sang in the choir and sometimes needed to be gently turned to face the front of the church." She continues: "One day, as the priest began

---

24. Killick and Cordonnier, *Openings*, 18.
25. Harkaway-Krieger, "Theology and Theories of Metaphor," 347.

the Great Thanksgiving Prayer, this woman spoke it with him, word for word. There was a sense of awe as we listened. She might not have been able to remember many things of her daily life, but with the thanksgiving prayer she spoke she seemed to enter into the experience of that sacred moment."[26]

From the discussion so far, it is possible to discern how, perhaps, a person in mid-stage dementia is continuing on their journey into God. Taken as a whole, there is no reason to see this as somehow a fall from full discipleship, a loss of spiritual meaning, or a diminishment of the person's faith: on the contrary, a good argument could be made from the teachings of Jesus in the Gospels that the appeal of the gospel and our response is more by means of the intuition and emotions, through metaphor and symbol, than by means of the discursive intelligence, through words and logic. We can see potential spiritual struggles along the way, as the believer loses touch with some of the discursive and credal landmarks of the faith; as they lose some control over their own emotions; as they have to learn to be more dependent on others. We can also see how a new and potentially frightening territory is opening up, as symbols take on a freshness, vibrancy, uncontrollability and salience in the life of faith. But there is also a hope, potentially some new insights into the presence of the Spirit, and a peace in trusting God.

Returning to the story of my mother with which I began the chapter, we can see that trust being acted out in her suggestions of prayer, that symbolization in the way she adopted the postures and intonations of prayer even though the language she was using made little formal sense. The movement of the heart in trust of God and surrounded by people with whom she has an emotional connection is clear enough to see. It is borne out in Julie Simpson's patient, detailed ethnographic study of people with "advanced" dementia in a care home context, whose ability to communicate and conceptualize was significantly impaired but who still had, she concluded, a vibrant spiritual life:

> Rather than coming to a place of "narrative foreclosure," defined as the person having no further possibilities for meaningful engagement, nothing to look forward to, and nothing to add to one's storied-life (Bohlmeijer et al. 2011), the person discovers fresh opportunities to express and enact their voice . . . in being together with others, and/or enjoying one's solitude, and connecting with meaningful activities and relationships, the spiritual dimension of

---

26. MacKinlay, "Journeys," 34.

each person with advanced dementia continues to be nurtured. The person continues to find meaning, purpose, and self-worth in the present.[27]

The fact that I was embarrassed and slightly irritated by my mother's expression of faith, by being cajoled to sit down and put my hands together while my mother repetitively prayed snatches of phrases without sentences, with words that to me did not "make sense," is perhaps an example of the sort of sickness that Symeon the holy fool was perceived as addressing. As a "respectable," sophisticated, educated Christian, for me the purpose of the words was their formal meaning: words of prayer needed to be clear to address the Word of God. I was overlooking the role of the words as metaphor, as opening to the mystery of God in their very inability to make the meaning of prayer clear; as being, in the eyes of God, about as meaningless as all the rest of our words and their trivial attempts to capture God's glory. And I was missing the gestures, the positioning, the body language, the emotions, the togetherness: all the other ways in which the grace of God was at work in the imponderable manifestations of the ecclesial body of Christ.

Perhaps (returning to the words of Pope Francis) people living with mid-stage dementia have to "invent it themselves" as the regulated meanings and clearly defined practices in which their discipleship has grown give way to a world of flat immanence and wildly unregulated, emotionally charged metaphor. And perhaps it is we who are blind to the commitment, the creativity, the courage with which individuals remake their spirituality, remain attentive to the promptings of the Christ into whose likeness they seek to be conformed. We can glimpse that world of faith and meaning, given enough attention and care. Julie Simpson encounters the same reaching for transcendence in some of the participants in her ethnographic study even as the last words are disappearing, as in this unedited extract from "Naomi":

> All I wonder. God! I still, I still, I still, I still . . .
> You're love. You're love . . .
> Well, that's wha . . . wein this worl, worl, worl . . .
> why we're in this worl, worl, worl![28]

---

27. Simpson, *"I Still,"* 208. Quotation from Bohlmeijer et al., "Narrative Foreclosure."
28. Simpson, *"I Still,"* 228. See also Collicutt, "Spiritual Awareness," 25.

However, it is harder to see how that understanding, that faith is at work and expressed as the middle stage of dementia gives way to the later stage, when speech is lost or very limited, and when a person's interaction with the people and world around them are growing fainter and less comprehensible. Here there is much less to go on, and we have to turn more explicitly to what we can learn from mysticism and theology. By faith, we maintain that God does not desert us in the depths of loss and pain, but is then most present to us; so the challenge is to find a way of conceptualizing this stage as a consummation of our discipleship rather than its destruction. As Robert Davis, looking forward to this stage in his own dementia, puts it,

> Perhaps the journey that takes me away from reality into the blackness of that place of the blank, emotionless, unmoving, Alzheimer's stare is in reality a journey into the richest depths of God's love that few have experienced on earth. Who knows what goes on deep inside a person who is so withdrawn? At that time, I will be unable to give you a clue, but perhaps we can still talk about it later in the timeless joy of heaven.[29]

The problem is that we do not easily find the tools and concepts that will allow us to think this thought. We want to say, with Teilhard de Chardin, that "when the painful moment comes in which I suddenly awaken to the fact that I am losing hold of myself and am absolutely passive in the hands of the great unknown forces that have formed me; in all those dark moments, O God, grant that I may understand that it is you (provided only my faith is strong enough) who are painfully parting the fibers of my being in order to penetrate to the very marrow of my substance and bear me away within yourself."[30] But it is not clear what it would mean to say that God is penetrating "to the very marrow of my substance." So the journey of the Christian disciple through dementia has some more to teach us, and this will be the subject of the next chapter.

---

29. Davis and Davis, *My Journey*, 120.
30. Teilhard de Chardin, *Milieu Divin*, 89–90.

7

Mum's last day
Does the flesh pray?

Daphne was an articulate, vivacious and intelligent woman, a lifelong Baptist with a keen theological mind; and on the day of her death, she got on her knees by the side of her bed. This apparently commonplace activity was remarkable because, by that stage, the woman who Daphne had been seemed to have already slipped away. By the time Daphne died, she was confined alternately to a hospital bed and a wheelchair, and appeared to have lost the capacity for purposive activity. She did not show signs of any awareness of her surroundings or of other people, and she had lost the ability to communicate by speech or gesture. But on the morning of her last day, Daphne somehow managed to get out of her bed unaided. Her devoted husband found her kneeling on the floor and managed to get her back into bed, where she died peacefully a few hours later.

From a detached, clinical perspective it seemed clear that, at this stage in her dementia trajectory, Daphne lacked the self-awareness or conceptual capacity for intentional action: the movement was, perhaps, the agitation of a body in its final stage of life, or at best a reflex or habitual act lacking any purpose. As her son, at the time that was my own fixed opinion. But in the opinion of her husband (who was the person best-placed to interpret his wife's actions and intentions) Daphne was praying: aware of her own impending death, she made a prayer of her body and surrendered herself to her God.

In late-stage dementia, the attributes and behavior that we identified with the spiritual life of the middle stage disappear. Language, metaphor, social responsiveness, intentional movement, and possibly even emotion itself eventually either disappear or become unavailable to us to interpret, replaced by the "blank Alzheimer's stare." Theologically, this presents us with some puzzles. If we say that prayer requires a level of cognitive capacity that Daphne does not have, we must conclude that some people are incapable of prayer, that most fundamental of human responses to God, which raises the question of how they may meaningfully be said to be "in God." On the other hand, if we assert that Daphne was in fact praying, we must conclude that there is a form of prayer that is not dependent on our capacity for conscious, intentional action—or at least, not in a form that we can detect. Finally, if Daphne continues to be a theological subject throughout the course of her dementia, we must assume that she continues *in via* as a disciple, with the moral and spiritual struggles and graces that characterize the mundane life of the Christian, and so accept this period of her life as theologically significant.

Throughout this book, I have maintained that since a person living with dementia continues as a theological subject, and God continues to be God, their relationship is maintained to the very end despite any appearances to the contrary for "spirituality is part and parcel of what it is to be a person, qua human being in the world . . . and we may say that if PWD [a person with dementia] no longer has spiritual needs, they are no longer a person."[1] But Daphne's story presses these commitments to their limit, and requires us to think through the issues carefully. For if we conclude that Daphne must be praying on this her last day despite apparently lacking the capacity to do so, then we must find a way of understanding prayer and praying that is not dependent in the final analysis on intellectual cognition, or intentionality, or language, or awareness of the surrounding world.

Prayer in a time of dementia: Who is the Daphne who prays?

Before deciding the question of whether or not Daphne can be said to be praying we need to have some idea of what prayer is. There are of course many definitions of prayer, and, taken as a whole, it proves remarkably difficult to provide a single clear one; but in this case we can exclude the more

1. Hughes, *Thinking Through Dementia*, 205.

discursive models (prayer as a conscious address to God) and the more passive quietist ones (prayer as an infused gift of God) since neither addresses the presenting question of how Daphne might be said to be approaching God or responding to God in prayer as a theological agent with advanced dementia. We need a more existential definition, something like this:

> To show devotion in prayer is literally to seek a God, and to seek to establish a relation to this God, but without certainty that what is prayed to is indeed what the believer thinks it is, or that it is something at all. One could go even further and suggest, that the extent to which a God is present in a human life, is ultimately manifested in the praying act of devotion itself. For praying is an existential comportment in and through which man [sic] establishes a relation to what he holds to be divine, indeed, the mode in which this relation comes to presence, in all its precarious uncertainty.[2]

There are still some problems here, notably the concept of "seeking," which normally implies a formed mental intention that is then translated into purposeful action. But setting aside for now what "intention" might look like in late-stage dementia, we are left with a living relationship, or "precarious uncertainty." If we wish to assert that this relationship is maintained, we are left with a limited number of options.

First, we may say that Daphne is capable of a world of intentionality, understanding, and agency that is not visible to us but intact: what has changed is not her prayer life but her ability to communicate about it in ways we can understand. The difficulty with this approach is that, while by definition it is not possible to gain detailed insights from those who can no longer communicate, the witness of Christians in earlier stages of dementia (notably Christine Bryden and Robert Davis) indicates potentially profound changes taking place in their faith-life.[3] If we fail to take these changes seriously we are denying the reality and profundity of the faith-journey that is dementia, as well as denying the embodied intertwining of our faith life with the organic life of our bodies and brains.

Secondly, we might say that Daphne is incapable of a relationship to God, but that her "spirit is held safe in the Lord," who is sovereign. As we have seen, this strategy is widely adopted in the literature,[4] but has some real problems in its unrefined form because, in appearing to safeguard our

---

2. Ruin, "Saying the Sacred," 292.
3. Davis and Davis, *My Journey*; Williams, *God's Not Forgotten Me*.
4. E.g., McKim, *God Never Forgets*.

understanding of God's sovereignty and Daphne's dignity "before God," it denies her capacity as a *partner* in the relationship, and so erases her as a theological agent who can respond to God. We cannot divide Daphne into an eternal essence that is somehow immune to the changes that her body and mind are undergoing and a suit of meat that is deteriorating. We are created material beings: if the whole of Daphne is not in a prayerful relationship to God, then none of her is.

A third and more subtle approach would be to see Daphne's life and intention as integrated over time, so this habitual action has a sort of ingrained intentionality. We may consider that the history, choices, relationships, and emotions accumulated through a faithful life are not simply erased but persist in diffused and extended form in an embodied life. I have developed this theme elsewhere[5] and it has some potential here. However, it will be necessary to show that Daphne's action is not just an attenuated echo in procedural memory of behavior that may once have had meaning, but represents a response here and now: we want to understand the *kairos* of prayer for Daphne, not the *chronos*. In the words of John Swinton:

> If I believed the story which tells me that such incidents are nothing more than remnants that manifest the continuing presence of procedural memory, I could rationalize these moments as just part of the person's condition. . . . But I don't believe in that story. In the story I choose to believe in, *something actually happens*, something that transcends and resists reduction to procedural memory. . . . What goes on in our bodies is not epiphenomenal to who and what we are. Our bodies cannot be separated from our minds even when our memories and intellectual abilities appear to be abandoning us. Our bodies remember things, and that memory is not without meaning.[6]

Taking these limitations seriously, we need to "stretch" our conception of prayer to open up some new possibilities. This will mean we need to root our account of prayer in the here-and-now of Daphne's response to God, as a whole person. We therefore have to be rooted in the phenomenology of the event before us: what is Daphne doing as she takes to her knees, and in what sense may we understand it as prayer? Even if Daphne is not consciously aware of an intention to pray or in possession of the language

---

5. Kevern, "Spirituality and Dementia."
6. Swinton, *Dementia*, 245–46.

in which to express it, can we say, nevertheless, that her created flesh prays in this moment?

Praying in the flesh

If we want to affirm that people living in the late stage of dementia may also pray, we need to develop a fuller picture of how the non-cognitive, non-verbal body may also be understood as responding to God, how a prayerful response to God may be understood as diffused through the "flesh" of the person living with advanced dementia. This will entail expanding our understanding of the language of prayer, to encompass the ways in which the physical body may possibly be oriented toward the divine. Can it be said that our body, in its physical, organic, prelinguistic form, has a spiritual status before God alongside our conscious subjectivity?

Although I am not aware of any comprehensive study of how prayer and the flesh of the body may be related, there is some support for the notion that there *is a relationship* from a number of different perspectives. For example, it has been observed that "spiritual" concepts seem to be expressed in bodily terminology across a wide range of language groups, notably in the Semitic languages of the Hebrew Bible and their Greek parallels in the New Testament. "Most, if not all, of the core concepts of the Old Testament involve a double-aspect conceptualization of the world. For example, breath and spirit are different aspects of the same thing. Heart is both a part of the body, but also a centre of human feeling and understanding."[7] This implies that, rather than our "spirituality" existing separately and being expressed in the language of physical metaphors, our responses to God start off as physical sensations or actions before they are reflected on and developed theologically. Physicality and spirituality seem entangled from the start, and "the fact that historically independent languages have the same linkages between physical and inner meanings suggests that they reflect how earlier humans actually saw things, and are not just some inventive use of words. It seems that these double-aspect linkages in our language reflect some deep reality rather than being a human invention."[8]

From a different literary perspective, this widely observed entanglement of bodily and spiritual senses of language is developed into the basis for a general theory of the emergence of consciousness in Julian Jaynes's

7. Watts, *Embodied Spirituality*, 89.
8. Watts, *Embodied Spirituality*, 90.

extraordinary work, *The Origin of Consciousness in the Breakdown of the Bicameral Mind*.[9] At the heart of the book is a close reading of *The Iliad*, which Jaynes uses to develop his idea that until relatively recently, there was much less distinction between thought, emotion, and physiology: when an ancient author stated that "my heart leapt within me" they meant exactly that, and perhaps ascribed it to the action of a god, with the notion of a separate, emotional and rational "inner self" emerging only as written language developed. Regardless of whether Jaynes's broad theory is accepted or not, he has made an important point here: that there is nothing "natural" in the way we think of ourselves as cognitive selves detached from the body, using cognition and language as the route to God. Before we begin the process of abstraction in language, the body already has a way of relating to God.

Furthermore, the "language of the body" seems to exist prior to words and constructs the deep structure of our religious universe. For example, it has been found that postures influence the degree to which we interpret events as miraculous, and the adoption of a low-power posture seems correlated with feelings of religiosity.[10] The body, it seems, has a religious language "hard wired" into it, and this may even provide the rudiments for a recognizable theology. Louis-Marie Chauvet neatly summarizes its key dimensions in *Symbol and Sacrament*: "Nothing can become significant for us without becoming invested by the body with the primordial schemes that are inherent for it."[11] As he goes on to say, God is invariably represented by an upright posture indicating a vertical axis, as "height" or "depth." Ethical decisions by contrast follow a left-right schema, as rightness (*sic*) is opposed to "sinisterness," both leftness and wrongness. History is laid out in the third dimension, with the future typically "before" us and the past "behind" us. The language of consuming, soiling, warmth are similarly ubiquitous in our spirituality and our theologies, denoting notions such as comfort, blessing, worthiness, cleansing, sustenance, healing, and curse. All these correlations show us that the language of the body is not secondary or metaphorical but "indicate an *existential topography which is constitutive of the internal structure of the human being.*"[12]

---

9. Jaynes, *Origin of Consciousness*.
10. Watts, *Embodied Spirituality*, 82.
11. Chauvet, *Symbol and Sacrament*, 148.
12. Chauvet, *Symbol and Sacrament*, 149 (original emphasis).

There is, then, a case in principle to conclude that "the flesh prays" in the way in which our response to sacredness is shaped and given its language by the body itself. Studies in linguistics, literature, and psychology all converge to suggest that the architecture and language of prayer may be inseparable from the structure and processes of the body.[13] However, this line of enquiry can in itself only take us as far as a sort of "natural theology" of prayer, a possible explanation for how prayer is conceivable to us as arising from physical processes, and why we are led through the experience of the body to some kind of spiritual response to something transcendent. It is an important step, challenging the assumption that the body can provide us only with metaphors for the soul's response to God taking place purely at a disincarnate spiritual level. However, we are seeking to understand whether and how Daphne is responding to a *particular* God, the God of her lifelong Baptist faith and discipleship. For this, it will be necessary to place the praying body in the context of the salvation history within which it is redeemed and sanctified, and to ask how her body, her flesh, is related to the body of the Incarnate Word. That is, we will need to supplement this phenomenological account with a theological one.

Graced flesh, praying flesh

Our guide for this stage of the exploration is Emmanuel Falque, who made an appearance in the earlier chapter on the sacramental body of Christ. Falque has been a key figure in what has been termed the "theological turn" in French phenomenology,[14] an upsurge in interest in the way in which close observation of religious phenomena may deepen our understanding of God.[15] His particular lifelong concern has been to recover the significance of the organic, fleshly and physical body and its experiences for theology, as "on the one hand, our passions and impulses, and, on the other hand, our biological and chemical nature, our concrete 'flesh and bones.'"[16] It is a concern that he has developed and extended in successive works, with his latest engaging most intensely with what it means for the body of

---

13. Hughes, Louw, and Sabat, *Dementia*; Fuchs, "Embodiment and Personal Identity in Dementia."
14. Janicaud, "Theological Turn."
15. Falque, *Crossing the Rubicon*.
16. Gschwandtner, "Corporeality, Animality, Bestiality," 2.

the incarnate and resurrected Christ to be, in all its carnality, a biological body.[17]

Running through this body of work is his working out of the claim that, in the incarnation, God becomes related to humanity "body to body" (*corps à corps*),[18] and that, consequently, our relatedness to God can best be understood through an intertwining of phenomenology and theology. To anticipate the argument I will be developing subsequently, we may be able to say that since the Son shares in the same flesh as Daphne, and since they can be related *corps à corps*, Daphne encounters the God she knows theologically in and through her embodied experience irrespective of her cognitive or linguistic capacity. But to state the conclusion thus baldly is to race through a number of steps that need to be examined in more detail: we need to see how the statement stands up to theological scrutiny, but also explore more fully what it might *mean*, for Daphne, for those who care for the faith of people living with advanced dementia, and for our understanding of prayer generally.

For this, the most appropriate vehicle is Falque's doctoral thesis, a study of the thought of early and medieval theologians published in English as *God, the Flesh, and the Other*. The second of the three parts, on the Flesh, traces a historically eccentric but theologically coherent route through the work of Irenaeus, Tertullian, and Bonaventure to build up a philosophy of the incarnation that bridges phenomenology and theology in a single vision. His primary concern here is to analyze phenomenologically how "the flesh" may be experienced in three modes: in relation to the human being; to the incarnate God; and to the human in relation to God;[19] but since our concerns here are somewhat different, we will trace a different path through his analysis. Briefly, the argument I will develop has three stages. First, that in becoming fully human, the Word prepares all flesh to share in divinity (Irenaeus); secondly, that the flesh responds to God in its own proper way, not simply as an "ark" or vehicle for consciousness (Tertullian); and finally, that the response of the flesh is marked and shaped by our intentional response to God, completed by the work of God's grace

---

17. Falque, *Wedding Feast*.

18. The term *corps à corps* is translated colloquially as "hand to hand," since it is most commonly encountered in the French term equivalent to the English "hand to hand fighting." However, the translation "body to body" is literally more correct and of more explanatory value here.

19. Gschwandtner, "Corporeality, Animality, Bestiality," 3.

(Bonaventure). We will then return to the question of Daphne's final day, and how its events can be understood as an instance of the body in prayer.

Irenaeus

At the heart of Irenaeus's theology is a chiastic structure summarized some decades later in Athanasius's most famous line, that Christ "assumed humanity so that we might become God."[20] This is not an alienation of the Word from the Godhead in order to suffer a fall into carnality, that is, the Word does not become less "godly" by becoming human. On the contrary, when the Word took flesh in the incarnate body of Christ, Christ effected a fulfillment of God's created order in its restoration as the "new Adam." As well as being the second person of the Trinity, Christ is "the image of the invisible God" in his flesh: the divine image that was perfectly presented in Adam and then marred is now returned to its intended glory in Christ. "If the first Adam (of Genesis) *prefigures* the second (the Word made flesh), it is because the second (Christ) *manifests* the full humanity of the first in his original formation (Adam drawn from the earth)."[21] There is therefore no fundamental discontinuity between our knowledge of our own flesh and our knowledge of God-as-enfleshed in Christ. We can know the Father in our flesh because in union with Christ it is restored to its status before the fall as *imago Dei*.

For Irenaeus, and in contrast with the "heretics" who, he says, treat the fall as a fall into materiality from an existence of abstract spiritual perfection, the flesh is the *reason* why humanity is uniquely graced and capable of becoming god-like: "The ontologically neutral thickness of the creation that confers on man a membership in animality and life in general is also the condition of the reception of grace. The Father is given to 'sons' who are capable of receiving him, and not to beings so oblivious of their creaturely ontological weightiness that they lose the originary pedestal that is theirs by virtue of their very being."[22] In Falque's reading of Irenaeus, then, "Organicity is not the source of the soul's alienation but is something with which it is intertwined and properly belongs. . . . The human being cannot be thought apart from this condition nor set in opposition against it, . . . we

---

20. Athanasius, *On the Incarnation*, 54.
21. Falque, *God, the Flesh, and the Other*, 121.
22. Falque, *God, the Flesh, and the Other*, 130.

are forever bound up in the medium of the flesh, which is always also the lived body."[23]

Christ, who is divine, becomes flesh; consequently, humanity, which is flesh, becomes divine. The perfect image of God becomes a human being; consequently, human beings are once again restored to the perfect image of God. This chiastic structure of incarnation and response is reproduced in a reversal of the relationships between fleshliness and language. If in the incarnate body of Christ the invisible Word of God of Judaism becomes visible and palpable, so the language of the human body becomes in turn expressive of the divine.[24] In the order of divine action, Word is prior to flesh; in the order of human response, flesh is prior to words. In Christ, God's originary creative Word becomes flesh for us; in our response, we find ourselves flesh-to-flesh (*corps à corps*) with the incarnate God, out of which issue our words of response. "'The Word was made flesh so that the flesh could become Word,' says Mark the Ascetic. . . . For us here this means precisely that the Word speaks even better in his flesh than in his speech, and it is by the flesh that his speech speaks."[25]

Two key insights can be gleaned from Falque's discussion of Irenaeus. First, since incarnation "goes all the way down," Christ's communion is with our flesh as fully as with our minds. Secondly, since our response to God originates from the Word-made-flesh, that response runs deeper than our ability to use language. Consequently, there can be no "partial communion" in Christ for those who are cognitively impaired, and the question is no longer *whether* Daphne can respond, but only *how* she responds in prayer.

Tertullian

In Falque's account, the particular contribution of Tertullian is (literally) to "flesh out" the theology of the incarnation of the Word developed by Irenaeus. As with Irenaeus, Tertullian is writing in opposition to a number of groups that were uncomfortable with the notion that "spiritual" things could be involved with the physical flesh, and so sought to understand Christ in non-physical ways. By contrast, Tertullian "attempts to feel the weight of the flesh of the incarnate Word in all its solidity and makes of his

---

23. Pappas, "Flesh," 84.
24. Falque, *God, the Flesh, and the Other*, 132.
25. Falque, *God, the Flesh, and the Other*, 120.

weight the defense against all our attempts to angelize the Incarnation."[26] His focus is intense and unwavering: "The central question of the *De carne Christi*, as it reflects on the modality of the flesh of Christ insofar as it informs the modality of our own flesh, is forcefully articulated in the following unique formulation: 'What sort of flesh [*carnis qualitatem*] can we and ought we recognize in the Christ [*debemus et possumus agnoscere in Christo*]?'"[27]

His answer is, explicitly and exhaustively, a physical one. Christ's body is made of the same substance as Adam's, of the same material as the created order, it is made of muscles, bones, nerves, and veins. However, where his account builds on Irenaeus's is by considering the body in act and motion, the body as *experienced* by Christ and by us. He asserts that Christ's actions and his experiences are precisely the same as ours, inasmuch as he is incarnate as one of us: as he moves through life, he experiences the parts of his body as flesh (esthesiology), and "by them he experiences in himself diverse kinestheses by virtue of which he constitutes the world (eating, drinking, weeping, etc.). The two *raisons d'être* of the flesh of Christ, according to the *De carne Christi*, namely, the kinesthesis and the esthesiology of the living, are therefore founded on one, since that which reveals his movement to us (kinesthesis) is at the same time that which attests to him as living (blood in his veins, the interlacing of nerves, etc.)."[28]

Two conclusions follow. The first is that for Christ, as for us, there is a kinesthetic response to the Father that derives from the flesh itself, prior to the expression in thoughts or words. "Does not the 'I can' of Christ's flesh described by the movements of his body . . . actually precede the intentionality of his 'I think'? The sensory lived experiences of his body . . . incarnate his body in the flesh (*es wird Leib*), inasmuch as by means of them, he constitutes the world."[29] Secondly, if this is the case, we become distracted if we seek to encounter Christ first in his words rather than his acts, and here Falque finds his support in the words of Hans Urs von Balthasar: "Even if 'flesh' here stands for 'man,' speaking is only one of the forms of activity of the being 'man.'"[30] Thus, at the points where Christ is most profoundly

---

26. Falque, *God, the Flesh, and the Other*, 143.
27. Falque, *God, the Flesh, and the Other*, 146.
28. Falque, *God, the Flesh, and the Other*, 156.
29. Falque, *God, the Flesh, and the Other*, 154–55.
30. Falque, *God, the Flesh, and the Other*, 164, quoting von Balthasar's words in *Glory of the Lord*, vol. 7, 142.

fulfilling his father's will, he is dumb: "Both the newborn in Bethlehem and the crucified man on Golgotha lack speech. Only the flesh speaks here." We can conclude that, because it is through action and experience in his flesh that Christ has plumbed the deepest reaches of our humanity, "the flesh is the hinge of salvation."[31]

It follows from these two points that our encounter *corps à corps* with the crucified and risen yet still physically embodied Christ takes place in actions: that physical movements themselves can be considered acts of communion and response to God without needing to be reduced to linguistic forms. We do not need to claim that "Daphne is trying to say . . . in words" in order to accept her action as a response to God: even if we understand her existence as reduced to the movement of blood in veins and the interlacing of nerves, she remains at the very "hinge of salvation" where the encounter takes place.

Bonaventure

Falque's passage through Bonaventure's work is broad ranging, taking in an analysis of the *Canticle of the Creatures* and a discussion of his doctrine of the spiritual senses; but the main focus of Bonaventure's work, for Falque's discussion, is his treatment of the stigmata of St. Francis, the spontaneous appearance in his hands, feet, and side of the wounds suffered by Christ at his crucifixion. As he recounts it, "Saint Francis of Assisi himself bore the carnal marks in his body (holes in his feet and hands and a pierced heart). Here, by way of the carnal experience of the divine, is established a new relation to God, to the body and to the world in general—a relation to which the Christian seems to be called by the voice of the incarnate and resurrected Word."[32]

In the first place, says Falque (drawing here on his treatment of the *Canticle of the Creatures*), the stigmata exemplify how God is manifested in the created order, symbolically or iconically: the symbolic constitutes "the act by which the 'holiness' of God takes shape, namely, by forms (parts, organs), location (and adornments), affects (anger, sadness, enthusiasm, intoxication), even kinestheses (sleep, vigilance). . . . The sensible therefore 'signifies' God himself, revealing his presence (icon) rather than returning

---

31. *Caro salutis cardo est*, Tertullian, *De resurrectione carnis* 8, 2, in Falque, *God, the Flesh, and the Other*, 165.

32. Falque, *God, the Flesh, and the Other*, 180.

to him in the mode of absence (trace)."[33] In short, Bonaventure considers Francis's stigmata as evidence about how God works in the world through our bodies, their sensations, their changes, and their parts. If God can induce the marks of wounds in the flesh of St. Francis, in our flesh God may at least be able to accomplish lesser feats: speaking to us directly through our bodies, bringing about physical changes that open us to God.

Secondly, in his "doctrine of conversion of the spiritual senses" Bonaventure maintains that this constant self-announcing of God in creation, in events and even in our own bodies, can be discerned by those who are faithful to Christ. It now becomes conceivable that the creator God may communicate directly through the senses with God's creation. "The definition of the spiritual senses show that even that which lives physically is capable of being spiritually converted . . . , for example, brother Francis who 'heard', in the call of the Crucifix of Saint Damien (1206), 'with the ears of flesh.' . . . It goes without saying that this does not mean that Francis heard a voice, but rather that what is lived spiritually is received carnally at the same time. . . . The realism of the incarnation imposes the thought of an encounter [*corps à corps*] of man and God even today."[34]

This doctrine then paves the way philosophically for an understanding of Francis's stigmata as a "limit experience."[35] As Bonaventure understands it, the stigmata are at one level a response to the constant meditation of Francis on the passion of Christ (engaging the body in prayer in the form of a cross as well as the emotions in tears of compunction) and at another a supernatural grace of the God whose marks are found throughout the created order. The very flesh itself is converted: "Now we reach the object of the present study: the 'conversion of the flesh' in Bonaventure ought to be seen as making visible, in the bodily experience of the saint, the very thing that was said and lived in the experience of the conversion of the senses . . . which discloses, even in a wounded and transformed flesh, the action of the Resurrected One in a possible but rare divine–human encounter [*corps-à-corps*]."[36]

The discussion of Bonaventure informs the dimension of our problem that is to do with Daphne's history and discipleship: the ways her lifelong Baptist devotion may have informed and shaped her response. In the first

---

33. Falque, *God, the Flesh, and the Other*, 181–82.
34. Falque, *God, the Flesh, and the Other*, 185.
35. Fuchs, Breyer, and Mundt, *Karl Jaspers' Philosophy*.
36. Falque, *God, the Flesh, and the Other*, 191–92.

place, we may speculate that the "conversion of the senses" engendered by Daphne's lifelong Christian discipleship had sensitized her to the traces of God's activity in her flesh and her environment: that, however impaired she was in her conscious awareness, she would have perceived in her flesh the imminence of her death and the presence of her God. Secondly, her life of religious practice would have shaped the responses of her body, providing her with a repertoire of physical responses that would include the gesture of kneeling.[37]

Daphne and the praying flesh

When Daphne takes to her knees on her last day, can she meaningfully be said to be praying? And if so how? We cannot know Daphne "from the inside": all we have is a movement, a positioning that incorporates some elements (breathing, touch, proprioception) that we know have some somatico-spiritual association with prayer at a prelinguistic level. Theologically, however, we may be able to say rather more. Drawing on Irenaeus, we may say that the natural mode of prayer to the Incarnate Lord is a fleshly one, *corps à corps*; and that the words that may arise as part of our prayer to God follow on from that encounter, are secondary to it. From Tertullian, we learn that the idiom of that prayer may be not so much in abstract concepts or linguistic constructions as in sensations and actions, a kinesthetic and esthesiological encounter that has its origins in the nerves, flesh, blood vessels, and even cells of our physical nature. Finally, from Bonaventure, we learn that the timing and form of that prayer (insofar as it is valid to talk of a nonlinguistic form) will have been shaped by a lifetime of devotion that has led to the "conversion of the senses." So although we cannot know for Daphne, any more than for anybody else, whether she is "really" praying in that moment, we can be cautiously confident that her cognitive impairment is no impediment to a true and prayerful encounter with the living God and that her life of faithfulness is pointing her toward an encounter *corps à corps*.

On the face of it, the story with which I began this chapter is a dismal one, an account of the last movements of a person in the last stages of her dementia and of her life. However, reviewing it in the light of the

---

37. There is a potential complication here, in that kneeling to pray is not typical of the Baptist tradition. However, it was and is central to the larger gestural vocabulary of the Western Christian tradition and would clearly be the most appropriate in this context.

incarnation has led us to some profound and evocative speculations. They suggest that the same Christ who governs the cosmos is, through that incarnation, present in all of humanity, a presence that is realized eternally and intimately in every cell of our being, *corps à corps*. The "deconstruction incarnate" that is the progression of dementia has laid bare an organic connection both to God and to the world that is not dependent on our capacities or our conscious, intentional responses but our very fleshliness. So the same incarnate body of Christ united to us spiritually also unites us bodily with all of creation, bringing us to fulfillment as representatives of the new Adam in our physical createdness. Daphne's fleshly body becomes the site of an encounter between God and God's physical creation, the site at which Christ, the new Adam, draws all things into union:

> Practically, the church as garden provides the space for solitude and contemplation particularly in the dung heap although I have not found much of this in the institutional church but from my friends, the "Dementing Priests" in the nursing home. Lost in Eden, they teach us more about our faith. They shepherd us, guiding us to recognize our illusions about life, and, most importantly, they administer to us a different sacrament of humility, accompanied by the music of the flowing river, the birdsong and the tree of death become the tree of life.[38]

This would be a satisfyingly positive note on which to end the exploration of faith in the company of people living with dementia. However, this account does not represent the apparent experience of every person of faith in the later stages of dementia. For many, the "last days" seem to be marked by extreme distress, suffering, isolation, and abandonment, and if this is the end of the story it is a tragedy. But it is *not* the end of the story, because for them, as for Daphne, at the end of the "last day" is physical death. To complete our understanding of the theological meaning of dementia, we must attempt to look past this "final frontier," to understand what it is that we will become when we become united in "one flesh" with Christ's body as his Bride. "The world, our world, must be broken *upwards* and *forward*, beyond and toward the End, and we must look *there* for our final redemption."[39]

---

38. Barclay, "Lost in Eden," 81.
39. Sonderegger, "Doctrine of Resurrection," 119.

8

Touching darkness, touching God
Dementia and the end of all things

I love the way Mel Bringle's hymn expresses the experience of dementia. The hymn's words, "When memory fades, and recognition falters . . ." shares what is happening to me. But the last verse expresses my hope: "Within your Spirit, goodness lives unfading. The past and future mingle into one. All joys remain, un-shadowed light pervading. No valued deed will ever be undone. Your mind enfolds all finite acts and offerings. Held in your heart, our deathless life is won." I sometimes think this might be read as, "our deathless life is one."[1]

I began this study with the Alzheimer's Society advert, and its claim that "With dementia, you don't just die once, you die again, and again." In subsequent chapters I questioned that account, and developed an understanding of the crucified Christ as one who accompanies us on the journey through dementia toward perfection in the image of God. Nevertheless, at a primal level, we experience dementia as a series of deaths, and the person we love seems much diminished at the end. We find in ourselves a desire to meet our loved ones on the other side of death; and while we hope for their

---

1. "Mark," in Horsburgh, *Impact of Holding Faith*, 223. The complete hymn can be accessed at https://www.junebergalzheimers.com/when-memory-fades-and-recognition-falters.

resurrection in Christ, we are driven to wonder what that resurrection will "look like."[2]

As well as at the personal level, at the theological level also, this is a useful question to ask. As I indicated at the end of the last chapter, to understand the theological significance of dementia we need to see the whole trajectory of the person's journey, not just from the inception of symptoms to their death but to our hoped-for resurrection. Specifically, I believe that my mother's experience of dementia will make sense from the point of view of the end of all things, and this belief provides the foundation for my belief that the period of her life lived with dementia was as rich with meaning as the rest of it. We can only understand Christ fully in the light of the eschaton—we have to know where his history is heading to perceive the meaning of the cross—and it may be the same for all of us. We may find that our lives, in all their jumble of apparent randomness and meaninglessness, will make sense when viewed from the perspective of God's eternal purpose for creation. In this chapter, I will unpack what that might mean, holding at the forefront the human, searching motive for our question: the desire that we will encounter each other, perfected in Christ, in eternity.

In the majority of contemporary theology, the practice of imagining life in heaven has rather gone out of fashion, and for good reasons: the Christian tradition is more focused on the eschaton as a this-worldly challenge, and trying to imagine a state in which both time and the physical world have been abolished or transformed is an unsettling business. Nevertheless, we cannot skirt this issue completely, if we are to locate a theological meaning in the experience of dementia. Thinking about "eternal life" is not just a matter of idle speculation, but conditions our understanding of what we are doing here and now. It "presses upon and transforms the character of present existence in ways which the doctrines of Christian life and ecclesiology must display and to which they must do justice."[3] Katherine Sonderegger (whose work has shaped this chapter) adds that there is an important imaginative component to this reflection on our understanding of the resurrected state: we need to "'fill it out', give it substantial form and heft, or allow it to work on and for us as an 'object of thought.' . . . The doctrine of Last Things cannot do real work in the Christian life, its gears

---

2. A wide range of terminology comes into play when talking about our future state, such as "the eschatological kingdom," "heaven," "resurrected body," and "perfected state." I have chosen not to be drawn into a discussion of their relative merits, and deploy my terms imprecisely in this chapter.

3. Zeigler, "Editor's Introduction," ix.

cannot engage, so long as the very color of Heaven is not made vivid before our eyes."[4]

Nevertheless, when thinking about somebody such as my mother, who spent her last years with dementia, there are some obstacles in the way of making heaven "vivid before our eyes," because it is no longer clear what we may hope for. For example, we may wish to assert that the period in which mum lived with dementia was an authentic expression of her journey toward union with God, and the relationship she had with her family and others during that period also had spiritual value. But we do not want to imagine that this is the entirety of God's purposes for her, or that she will spend eternity defined by dementia in this way. Will she be restored to a "perfect" state before the onset of dementia (and if so, at what age, in what state?), or will the dementia somehow continue to be part of who she is for eternity?

Resurrection and perfection

In some Christian traditions (such as some Black Pentecostal churches and the Jehovah's Witnesses), in popular devotion, and in "folk religion," there is a continuing rich tradition of imagining what life will be like in heaven, and what our loved ones may be doing there. At that human level, we may imagine a resurrected life that resembles the present one but idealized and extended indefinitely. We may imagine meeting our loved ones in heaven, all their injuries healed, and the marks of aging erased. We may imagine perfected individual bodies at an ideal age, continued relationships among spouses or parents and children.

This position is developed theologically in the work of Thomas Aquinas. Aquinas considers that the body will be fully restored physically, and he specifically concludes that parts such as entrails, hair, and nails will rise again in the resurrected body. Losses and deficits acquired in life (e.g., loss of a limb) are restored in the eschaton because the soul is the form, end, and cause of the body, which is its realization, something like a work of art.[5] Hence, imperfections accrued during life are irrelevant because they do not touch the soul. This is the understanding of bodily resurrection that, for most of us, best represents our assumptions and desires. We would want to rise healthy, strong, beautiful: our "best self," in the prime of life and as

---

4. Sonderegger, "Doctrine of Resurrection," 118.
5. Aquinas, *Summa Theologica*, Supplement, Question 80.

perfect as we can imagine. Heaven (or, perhaps, the new earth) would then be a place of endless fellowship in which fulfilled individuals with perfect bodies encounter each other in perfect peace and charity, for ever.[6] In this understanding, there would be no place for dementia: as it has recently been argued again by Terrence Ehrman, this view can understand disabilities only as privation, the lack of a good that, as members of God's good creation, people should have. It follows that, in the resurrected body, these deficiencies will be made good.[7]

There is a superficial attractiveness to this view, not least because it takes our instinctive desires for the "good life" and projects them forward into an idealized version of the present: it does not require of us too much imaginative work. But on further reflection, it raises some difficult questions. For example, is there a perfect age and state to which we should be returned? Perhaps the Aristotelian notion of perfect form as being a male in his thirties should be applied to all as the universal form possessed by the soul? If so, can we all expect to be resurrected in this form? Thomas Aquinas seemed to think so, as "human nature will be brought by the resurrection to the state of its ultimate perfection which is in the youthful age, at which the movement of growth terminates, and from which the movement of decrease begins."[8] Clearly this is an absurd conclusion—imagine meeting your children, parents, and grandparents simultaneously, all perfectly restored to about thirty years of age—but it points to the weakness in Aquinas' argument: that if the soul is unchanging over time and circumstance, none of the changes that take place over the course of a life can be treated as anything other than progress toward, or lapses from, an immutable template. It also goes against one of the core assumptions of this book, that a person living with dementia is no less themselves than they were at any other point in their lives and that the experience of dementia is telling us something important about what it is to be in the image of God. To simply

---

6. The Jehovah's Witnesses have developed a distinctive artistic tradition that attempts to visualize just such a perfected state that lends an instantly recognizable style to *Watchtower* publications. See, e.g., https://www.jw.org/en/library/books/learn-from-great-teacher-jesus/gods-peaceful-paradise-you-can-live-there/.

7. Ehrman, "Disability and Resurrection Identity." See also the detailed analysis of Aquinas's position in Waddell, "Thomas Aquinas."

8. Aquinas, *Summa Theologica*, Supplement, Question 81. However, he stops short of stating that all should be of the same height or sex, on the grounds that differences of height or sex are not defects in the same way.

treat it as a privation of the good is to thin human experience down and strip it of its theological richness.

So if we want to say that the whole of our life (including the period living with dementia) is worthy of redemption and resurrection, how may we appropriately imagine the resurrected body? A similar question has been pondered in disability theology in relation to a range of disabilities. In Nancy Eiesland's radical work on the *Disabled God*, Jesus's wounds are part of his resurrected body, summarized in a passage to which I alluded in chapter 3:

> Here is the resurrected Christ making good on the incarnational proclamation that God would be with us, embodied as we are, incorporating the fullness of human contingency and ordinary life into God. In presenting his impaired hands and feet to his startled friends, the resurrected Jesus is revealed as the disabled God. Jesus, the resurrected Savior, calls for his frightened companions to recognize in the marks of impairment their own connection with God, their own salvation. In so doing, this disabled God is also the revealer of a new humanity.[9]

Amos Yong follows Eiesland's lead to argue that, if we read the resurrection appearances through the lens of disability, we may conclude that the disabilities that are constitutive of our identity will be retained in our redeemed eschatological bodies. As Jesus's scars become, instead of marks of shame or loss, the signs of his identity and his glory, so in the eschatological body there may be a "transvaluation" of the marks of disability. He contends that the New Testament suggests that "some impairments are so identity-constitutive that their removal would involve the obliteration of the person as well."[10]

It is easy to see why a person who had been blind from birth might consider that their blindness was so central to their experience of the world that it makes no sense to imagine it gone in the eschatological body. But this argument would surely not apply in the same way to dementia: while we would want to say that the person is no less themselves in the period that they are living with dementia, we do not consider dementia to constitute their identity. So that raises a deeper question: which aspect(s) of their life and which times *are* "constitutive"? And what happens to the contingent non-constitutive ones?

---

9. Eiesland, *Disabled God*, 100.
10. Yong, *Bible, Disability, and the Church*, 121.

Developing Yong's line of thought, Maja Whitaker makes a similar distinction between "identity-defining" and "non-identity-defining" changes and disabilities. The resurrected body needs to have sufficient continuity with our mundane loved body to be "us," and yet transformed, so "the biological criterion of identity will persist post-resurrection in each individual, though the precise expression will be transformed from decay and weakness to flourishing and splendor in a manner about which we can only speculate."[11] This is useful in that it reminds us that, by definition, the transformation of the resurrected body is outside our frame of reference, but it still presents us with too strict a binary between the two types of disability. As she herself argues, there is a substantial class of characteristics (such as a double mastectomy) that fall somewhere in the middle; and what counts as potentially "identity-defining" will vary from person to person. In the case of dementia, few would claim that it was somehow identity-defining, but it does not follow that it has no significance for the resurrected life. The years lived with dementia as a defining feature of a person's daily life cannot be written off in this way.

The difficulties we encountered above suggest that we may be approaching the question from the wrong angle by starting with ourselves as individual subjects who each have an "identity" derived from a set of unchanging attributes held in isolation, which we anticipate being made complete at the general resurrection. There are two assumptions implicit in this line of thought that I want to question in what follows. First, there is the idea that our "identity" lies in being independent, self-contained images of God. As we noted in the discussion of the *imago Dei* in chapter 1, this is only one, rather impoverished, way to understand what makes us human, and it is not adequate to the task before us. Instead, I propose that we start from the identity of Christ himself. We have a foretaste of the glorified body of Christ in the eucharist, in which we encounter it in the *anamnesis* of Jesus's sacrifice, in the visible and ecclesial body of the Church, and in eating the consecrated elements that are the resurrected body and our participation in the eschatological feast. The question then becomes how, at the resurrection, our bodies share in *this* body.[12]

The second assumption is one in which the final goal is completeness, a sort of closure of the questions surrounding our mundane lives. We imagine that this fallen created order is one of lack and dependence, but that

---

11. Whitaker, "Perfected yet Still Disabled?"
12. Pope Paul VI, *Sacrosanctum Concilium*, para. 47.

we will all be individually fulfilled in the eschaton. By contrast, in a startling development, Sonderegger argues that we should imagine our future state as one of radical *incompleteness*, the naked acknowledgment that our completion lies only with and in God and the relationships with others. "In the Age to Come, all creatures, animate and inanimate, will manifest their *incompleteness*, their radical fragmentation and dependence on God alone. What believers long to see with the eyes of faith . . . is the utter contingency of nature upon the One Source of Life."[13]

In what follows I will explore what happens when we set aside these two core assumptions and imagine our resurrected life as one of radical incompleteness, dependence, and openness to God and each other. I will approach the question of our own eschatological hope by an exploration of two key biblical passages, addressing in turn our physical and social future, through the perspective of the physical and ecclesial bodies of Christ. To anticipate, the conclusion will be along these lines, which we already encountered in chapter 3:

> God is in solidarity with humanity at its most fundamental level, in its weakness and brokenness. This is not to romanticize weakness. Rather, here God reveals the divine nature as compassion not only by undergoing or suffering with human vulnerability, but also by raising it up into God's own being. . . . So instead of doing away with impairments and the capacity to suffer, redemption transforms vulnerability into a communion with God, prefiguring the final eschatological horizon to come, when all things will become so transformed.[14]

The physical body of Christ: Resurrection and the narrative of the self

Addressing the question of bodily resurrection in his first letter to the Corinthians, Paul argues that the model and firstfruits of our resurrected body are alike in Christ:

> Christ has indeed been raised from the dead, the firstfruits of those who have fallen asleep. For since death came through a man,

---

13. Sonderegger, "Doctrine of Resurrection," 122.
14. Reynolds, *Vulnerable Communion*, 18.

the resurrection of the dead comes also through a man. For as in Adam all die, so in Christ all will be made alive.[15]

There is an echo here of a theme that Paul himself develops in Romans 5, but is most extensively elucidated by Irenaeus in his doctrine of "recapitulation" (*anakephalaiōsis*): that Christ as the new Adam re-lives the life and destiny of the first Adam, but without sin, and so opens an uncorrupted way to union with God for those who follow in his way.[16] Christ is the head of a column, a procession of the saints treading the road back from the fall of Adam toward the New Jerusalem. Consequently, all that happens to human beings on the road to perfection in God is part of that perfection, and in the words of St. Catherine of Siena, "All the way to heaven is heaven, because Christ is the way."

The doctrine of recapitulation suggests that our whole life "in time" is gathered together in Christ's work as the new Adam. We may imagine that all of the "selves" we have been, all the attributes that at different points have contributed to them (including the experience of dementia), will be gathered up into eternity.[17] However, we must not be misled into thinking of it as a simple *continuation* (or idealization) of our present state; and Paul argues for the importance not just of *time* in our understanding of human beings but also the central importance of *discontinuity*:

> But someone will ask, "How are the dead raised? With what kind of body will they come?" How foolish! What you sow does not come to life unless it dies. When you sow, you do not plant the body that will be, but just a seed, perhaps of wheat or of something else. But God gives it a body as he has determined, and to each kind of seed he gives its own body. . . . So will it be with the resurrection of the dead. The body that is sown is perishable, it is raised imperishable; it is sown in dishonor, it is raised in glory; it is sown in weakness, it is raised in power; it is sown a natural body, it is raised a spiritual body.[18]

---

15. 1 Cor 15:20–22.

16. Irenaeus, *Against Heresies* 3.22.

17. For as Boethius puts it, eternity is not the extension of time from a present into an indefinite future but "grasps and possesses wholly and simultaneously the fullness of unending life, . . . lacks naught of the future, and has lost naught of the fleeting past; and . . . must keep present with itself the infinity of changing time." Boethius, *de Cons. Philos.* prose VI, quoted in Greggs, "Order and Movement," 3.

18. 1 Cor 15:35–38, 42–44.

Expanding this metaphor, we may say that our progress through life (including dementia) brings us to the point of maturation as a "seed": in that sense all the events of life are retained in the person we have become, and the period of life lived in the presence of dementia is as integral to the person we are to become as all the others. All of life contributes to the maturation of the "fruit" that is to come, but does not determine its form.

Some sense of the meaning of this tension between continuity and discontinuity can be discerned in the Gospel narratives of the appearances of Christ in his resurrected body. Repeatedly, Jesus appears initially unrecognizable by those close to him, until he introduces a narrative detail that establishes continuity with his earthly self. Thus, for example, there are moments of disclosure when he calls Mary's name in the garden; when he enacts a characteristic miracle for those who had returned to fishing; when he eats a morsel of fish with them; when he breaks bread on the road to Emmaus; and most tellingly, when Thomas puts his hand into the wounds.

The picture here is of both transformation and continuity, but in terms of actions and memories rather than of fixed characteristics (with the possible exception of the Thomas incident). For us too, because there is no resemblance between the seed and the resurrected body, we cannot claim that the personal attributes of any particular period (childhood, disability, dementia, parenthood) somehow constitute our core "identity" in the resurrected body: all those historical stages with their physical characteristics are caught up into a glorified body that is of a different order and "the finality of the resurrection entails, as we have seen, that the life of the world to come is not a continuation of this life but a consummation of it."[19] Our true, final, and perfected "identity" will derive not from our attributes or history but from our gathering into a final, unmediated communion with God in Christ: "the glory and power of the resurrection body will derive not from some able-bodied ideal of perfection but from its mediating the gracious activity of God."[20]

I have argued that attempts to identify what a person will be after the resurrection are wrongly directed because our "identity" will not be defined by a set of characteristics that are somehow our independent possessions. Instead, we will be defined by our relationship to Christ in a position of absolute openness to and dependence upon the grace of God. In the case of my mother, for example, her resurrected "identity" cannot be understood

19. Ticciati, "Resurrection."
20. Yong, "Disability," 18.

as either having the characteristic signs of dementia or not, since characteristics will not be "had" in that sense. In the light of the resurrection of the body, the meaning of the past and the present is only to be found in a future that we cannot conceive, that is related to our present as fruit to seed. We need to let go of individual subjectivity in the way we have come to understand it, and individual agency as a personal property, since these belong to a mundane and finite order that is passing away.

Resurrection and the social self

If our individual lives are recapitulated and transformed beyond recognition in the general resurrection, the question arises of how, if at all, our social relations are preserved or transformed. As I argued in the opening chapter, our personhood may be understood as socially conferred and socially preserved: Does it make any sense to talk of my continuation as an individual if the set of social relations that defines and constitutes them is no longer in place? This question is addressed by Brian Brock, who argues that the question of how disability contributes to the resurrected body is wrongly put, since it treats the eschatological body in isolation whereas what is resurrected is the eschatological *community*. Disabilities can and should be incorporated into an eschatological community in which all are at ease with their social identities.[21]

This is an important corrective to the treatment of disabilities as the properties of individual bodies and a reminder that, in the case of dementia, as with other chronic conditions, the experience and categorization are as much about a dysfunctional community as a dysfunctional body. But it implies a character to the eschatological community that is a transformation of the present-day Church, not merely its extension. In the first place, the eschatological community must necessarily include a much wider range of people than those who constituted the earthly Church, because if our social selves are to be resurrected, those networks that shape and maintain us must also be resurrected, including all those currently outside the Church. This suggests something close to a universal resurrection. Secondly, these networks cannot be considered simply as collectivities (or "congregations") of individuals, since the relationships of the community as a whole will be transformed as the individuals themselves are. As with the discussion of the

---

21. Brock, *Wondrously Wounded*. See also the discussion of his approach in Gosbell, "Space, Place."

resurrection of individuals, here we are making a mistake if we start with the present reality and seek to extrapolate from it into a higher, more glorious version of the same: instead, we must start with the resurrection and glorification of Christ and understand the resurrection of social networks from that perspective.

In order to explore these themes in greater depth, we can turn to another passage that considers the eschatological hope of resurrection, but this time from the perspective of the collective, rather than the individual:

> For he chose us in him before the creation of the world to be holy and blameless in his sight. In love he predestined us for adoption to sonship through Jesus Christ, in accordance with his pleasure and will—to the praise of his glorious grace, which he has freely given us in the One he loves. In him we have redemption through his blood, the forgiveness of sins, in accordance with the riches of God's grace that he lavished on us. With all wisdom and understanding, he made known to us the mystery of his will according to his good pleasure, which he purposed in Christ, to be put into effect when the times reach their fulfillment—to bring unity to all things in heaven and on earth under Christ.[22]

In Ephesians 1, and unlike 1 Corinthians 15, Paul is not addressing the behavior and thinking of individuals, but the nature of the Church as the sign and foretaste of the eschatological body of Christ, in which "all things" will be brought to unity under Christ. Interestingly, the operative term in verse 10 is *anakephalaiōsasthai*, a variant of the same word used by Irenaeus of Christ's "recapitulation" of time, but here it refers to the gathering-together in Christ of the multiplicity of "all things" in the created order, and to Christ as the Head (*kephalos*) of that body.[23] Drawing on our consideration of 1 Corinthians 15, we may say that the earthly Church is related to the final unity of "all things" as the seed is to the fruit, gesturing to an eschatological reality that it shares, but does not fully embody: we are able to assert that the relationships, the social identities comprising the Church, will not disappear at the eschaton but be gathered up into the eschatological *anakephalaiōsis* under the headship (however construed) of Christ, for "we creatures, in truth, are *organically* and metaphysically intertwined and

---

22. Eph 1:4–10.

23. The root meaning of the term is "to summarize," and so to recapitulate and also to summarize under a single heading. The only other use in the New Testament is in Romans 13:9, referring to the golden rule as "summing up" the commandments.

dependent; we need each other as lungs need air."[24] Far from being made somehow perfect and independent in an individual resurrected body, this interdependence will become manifest and complete: "My completeness in this life will be broken open to the radical need, dependence and relation of the Spiritual Life."[25]

Reflecting scripturally on what it might mean to be resurrected into a social context has brought us to a similar conclusion to that of the previous section. Like our personal individuality, our social self is destined to die and to be resurrected, transformed. The character of that transformed and resurrected body is not one in which I "possess" or can manage my social identity, but one of radical dependence, in which I am defined by a social network that is itself defined by and dependent on the headship of Christ. It follows that the features that characterize and shape my social interactions—including perhaps dementia and the marginalization that "malignant social psychology" inevitably leads to—become irrelevant in the new social order under Christ's headship, as our relations to the head restructure all the others.

Perfection revisited

We began this chapter by considering what sort of a resurrected life might be imagined for somebody whose last days were marked by dementia, in the first section exploring how it might continue to be part of their individual and social "identity" and what we might hope for; I concluded that the starting point needed to be not the individual but the resurrected Christ. In the following two sections, I unpacked this conclusion through an analysis of two Christological passages, and argued that, from a Christocentric perspective, the question of what happens to my "identity" was wrongly put. If my personal identity is only defined and maintained by my relationship of radical dependence on Christ as the firstfruits of the new creation; and if the social network that defines me can only subsist in Christ under whose headship are gathered all things into unity; then the questions of personal attributes or social positioning become irrelevant or misleading. In this transformed kingdom, all times in the personal narrative, all relations in the social matrix, are brought to a single conspectus in Christ.

---

24. Sonderegger, "Doctrine of Resurrection," 124.
25. Sonderegger, "Doctrine of Resurrection," 125.

In the light of these reflections, it appears that the eschatological resurrection of the body has some startling features that set it apart from any dreams of a simple extension of the present order into the future. In the first place, I have argued that resurrection makes no sense except as having its origins and end in the crucified, risen, and glorified body of Christ. Within the history of that body is recapitulated and redeemed all of human history, including the histories of each one of us, in narratives that alone can give meaning to the whole. To be made subject to the reign of the resurrected body of Christ is therefore to surrender control of the self-narrative, of our derived and shadowy attempts at meaning-making. Similarly, under the headship of the resurrected Christ are gathered all things in heaven and on earth, in a manner that is foreshadowed in the ecclesial body of Christ and yet outstrips it both in quality and scope. The restored relationships it foreshadows are fulfilled as we are made members of an eschatological community that has no boundary and no outside. For the new to arrive, the old order must be swept away.

The analysis so far provides some reassurance that, for a person whose final days were defined by dementia, their struggles are neither determinative of their "identity" from an eschatological perspective nor completely irrelevant. This however is a negative finding, and there is a more positive one to be nurtured into view from the discussion above. It rejects the view that our deficient and defective lives will somehow be completed and returned to us in a perfected state, and instead suggests that our eternal destiny is to be permanently and definitively *incomplete*, insofar as we will subsist only in radical communion with and dependence on God in Christ. The order of salvation history is not from an incomplete created order to a completed eschatological one, but from a complete (if wayward) created order to an eschatological one of radical openness and need. Rather than looking for a vision of resurrected bodies complete in themselves, we need "a doctrine of resurrection, in which creation, perfectly complete in its own terms, is broken open to show its incompleteness and completed by its dependence on God alone. Self-sufficient and self-enclosed creatures are laid bare both in their radical dependence on God and in their essential relatedness to one other. A good, original completeness is thus superseded by an eschatological incompleteness which outstrips the original."[26] Our incompleteness is not assuaged, but becomes the basis for its fulfillment in relationship to God and others; and according to this picture, the general

---

26. Ticciati, "Resurrection," referencing Sonderegger, "Doctrine of Resurrection."

resurrection is not the inauguration of some kind of individualized perfection, the institution of a fantasy theme park of personal joys. It is the final disclosure of our individual incompleteness, the breaking-open of our inturned lives and instrumental social relations, to a naked acknowledgment that we can only be completed in God and in each other. It is when our personal narratives and identities are opened out and surrendered to be completed as members of Christ's body that, in our radical incompleteness, we find fulfillment.

This brings us back to a theme that has recurred throughout the book as a sort of organizing principle. We have encountered Christ as paradoxically known in the breaking-open of his body on the cross; as the historical church, which becomes the ecclesial body of Christ when it is broken open by those who disrupt its margins and overspills them; as the sacramental body in the broken bread of the eucharist; in the breaking-open of language in the fractured metaphors of faith to let in the light of the Word; as the heavenly body of Christ *corps à corps* in the breaking-open of our own bodies in late-stage dementia. In each of these situations, we have recognized Christ at work at the point where determinate "identities," whether individual, cognitive, or collective, are broken down and dissolved.

What, then, can we say of the experience of dementia, and what does it say to us of our future in God? In the light of the discussion above, we can no longer say that the process of dementia is a progressive loss of humanity, a falling-away from full personhood into a partial state in which the only hope is that God will eventually reverse it in the general resurrection, restoring us to full cognitive capacity. On the contrary: in the light of this analysis, the experience of dementia emerges as something more like a preparation for the life to come, an anticipation of the process of stripping that we will all have to undergo in order to be prepared for the transformative fullness of liberating and defining absolute dependence on our relationship to the glorified Christ for our identity. For those of us who believe in purgatory (and I confess I find this at best a difficult doctrine) it may be considered an anticipation of the process that we will all have to undergo in order to join the ranks of the saints. The losses and deficits, the bereavements and wounds of dementia are part of the fierce purgation that we must all experience on the journey to full incorporation into Christ. The very nakedness of the disease that Keck termed "deconstruction incarnate"[27] could be the preparation for grace, the moment of darkness before the eternal dawn.

---

27. Keck, *Forgetting*, 21.

Conclusion
Deconstruction incarnate and the Incarnate, deconstructed

> What, then, shall we say in response to these things? If God is for us, who can be against us? He who did not spare his own Son, but gave him up for us all—how will he not also, along with him, graciously give us all things? . . . Who shall separate us from the love of Christ? . . . For I am convinced that neither death nor life, neither angels nor demons, neither the present nor the future, nor any powers, neither height nor depth, nor anything else in all creation, will be able to separate us from the love of God that is in Christ Jesus our Lord.[1]

THIS BOOK STARTED WITH my mother's experience of dementia, and a few provoking questions that arose for me in response. Behind those questions were some basic assumptions that started me on this journey:

1. that the God mum had served all her life had not changed or abandoned her, but was accompanying her on her journey

2. that, equally, she remained a Christian disciple, and her faith remained intact, even as the dementia progressed

3. that, nevertheless, her dementia was not peripheral to her life in Christ but integral to it

What has arisen along the way as we have traced the implications of these commitments for our understanding of God, persons, and faith itself, has been speculative rather than critical, constructive rather than systematic. It is by no means the only route that could have been taken, and the

---

1. Rom 8:31–32, 35, 38–39.

conclusions to each chapter are not the only ones that could have been reached. But there is a logic in the way these relatively unassuming starting-points have opened up some rich themes in new ways; and in this final chapter, they deserve unpacking further.

The assertion that mum's personhood and faith remained intact even as dementia progressively eroded the ways in which she would once have embodied it in thoughts, words, and deeds raised the question of what a "person" is in the eyes of God, and how personhood is properly expressed. Resistance to the claim that dementia is a succession of small deaths, no more than the progressive loss of all that makes us human, brought us to the notion of our identity in the image of God. But because we had to recognize that, for all that, dementia *did* entail real losses of attributes that are typically associated with what it is to be human, we had to find a different way to think about the *imago Dei*. We found it in two related ways: in Comensoli's argument that to live in the image of God was to accept the unique life given by God to be lived; and in the recognition that the perfect image of God is Jesus Christ. These moves opened up a different set of questions about the personhood of somebody living with dementia. Instead of seeking to maintain their personhood by repeatedly affirming, against appearances, that they were still the same person "underneath," we could recognize that their personhood was, as with all of us, evolving in the unremitting flux of a life lived; because it is that life, given by God, in which it must necessarily take place.

Our search for the God who, in the face of dementia, is nevertheless constant and present, brought us to the notion of the "bodies of Christ." I argued that the constancy of God cannot be satisfied with a God who, in the face of profound forgetfulness, "always remembers" on our behalf; or one who, at the end of the ordeal, will be found waiting for us. If we are in the image of God when we live the life God has prepared for us, then it is in the midst of that life—with its losses, challenges, and deficits—that we will encounter God. This led us to the person of Christ as God Incarnate in our lives, and three modes of divine "presence to us" in what I termed the three bodies of Christ. First, we could say that Christ shared our physicality even to the point of acute delirium, and so embodied in salvation history the "deconstruction incarnate" we experience in dementia: we are not alone. Secondly, Christ is present as the ecclesial body, the Church, in the historical struggle between what the Church is called to be and the intermittent "malignant social psychology" of its historical institutions. Finally, Christ

Conclusion

is present to us in his resurrected and sacramental body, given for us to consume.

This brought us to consider how a period of life lived with dementia may nevertheless be one filled with theological meaning and Christian purpose. We needed to consider what it meant to be conformed to the likeness of God in Christ, without leaning on ideas of cognitive beliefs, intentional agency, or responsiveness to the world. This led us to the idea finally of conforming to the likeness of Christ as "touching God," an alignment *corps à corps* with the incarnate God: in the sacrament chewed and swallowed; in the intimacy of communion that we could observe opening up for some people as language burst out into metaphor and their dependence on the verbal and cognitive rules of communication was lessened; finally in the cells of my mother in her late-stage dementia, her very body "in touch" with the incarnate Christ.

Along the way on this journey, some other themes emerged organically that deepened the exploration. Chief of these was emptying, *kenosis*, as the route by which Christ could be "identified" and, in turn, the way in which our own true identity in the divine image emerged. So it was only when the physical body, mind, and even spirit of Jesus of Nazareth had been surrendered and systematically obliterated on the cross that, in Mark's account, the centurion can declare that he was, truly, (a) Son of God. His ecclesial body exists in history only as an actual, historical, social institution that remains open to corruption, faithlessness, and "malignant social psychology," one whose true identity as body of Christ frequently seems lost or obscured. And according to Marion, Christ is recognizable in the sacrament of the eucharist precisely in his humility, his hiddenness in the physical forms of bread and wine; one that draws forth from us an answering *kenosis* of self-abandon.

So this redemptive process of *kenosis* by which God becomes present to us then elicits an answering movement by means of which we become fully ourselves, in God. Jimmie G, the "Lost Mariner," is found when he gives himself over to the power of God in the sacrament; when he loses himself in that moment. Similarly, the institutional church shines forth as the ecclesial body of Christ at the point at which it abandons the boundaries that define its social identity to include the outsider, the strange and the unpredictable, embodied in the "holy fool" tradition. Finally, we all become ourselves when we accept the stripping—of our cognition, our agency, our ordered psychological lives—that was embodied once in the passion of

Christ and is embodied in the process leading "from cognition, through emotion, into spirit" and so to my mother's last day.

If "all the way to heaven is heaven, because Christ is the way" then we should not be surprised (although I was) to find a similar theme emerging in the last chapter. Abandoning the idea that we were to be restored to our "best selves" as independent individuals conforming to a template of perfection, the only way it was possible to think of eschatological completeness was in terms of radical openness and dependence: of the resurrected self as one that is incomplete in itself and exists in a perfected state only as completely open to and dependent on the resurrected Christ and the network of relationships within which we have our social being.

Bringing these two themes—of *kenosis* and eschatological incompleteness—together, and bringing them to bear on our thinking about dementia, leads to some unsettling notions. From the perspective of our final destiny as radically incomplete, dementia does not appear as a monstrous distortion of or sickness in our humanity, but something more like a step on the way to our transformation. Although initially shocking, at one level this is trivial: we are surely all used to the idea that our minds, like our bodies, will undergo "deconstruction" on the road to a future glory, that every part of us will die. But if, in dementia, somebody is progressively handing themselves over in trust to the God who is present *corps à corps* at the heart of their being, perhaps we should be looking to them as "spiritual pioneers" and inspirations on the road that we are all destined to travel.

To return to the question from the first chapter, perhaps we dread dementia so profoundly because the journey of a person through their dementia enacts for us, in "slow motion" as it were, the stripping away of self that we must all undergo on one side or the other of our physical death; because we see laid out before us the *kenosis* we will have to undergo on the way to our own resurrection. But if this book has laid out, often in rather graphic detail, the losses and darkness that can accompany the journey through dementia, I hope it has also made clear the basis for our hope in God: a God who accompanies us through every step along the way, whether recognized and acknowledged or not, not at a respectful distance but organically connected to us, intimately "in touch" with us.

The way in which the metaphor of "touching God" emerged and kept reemerging through the course of this book was a surprise, and in some ways a rather uncomfortable one. The idea of Christians touching has lately taken on an unclean odor, soiled by association with the recurrent acts of

Conclusion

sexual and physical violence perpetrated and colluded with by generations of church dignitaries over several decades. In religious circles, touch has become the pariah sense, the "untouchable" term, and we are all the poorer for it. For there is no other way to express the intimate closeness of God in Christ, or God's continuing communion across the span of our earthly life from our emergence out of a rudimentary ball of cells until our last breath, even in the midst of the destruction of our conscious self by dementia. Touch is the first of our senses to develop and the last to leave, the most immediate and omnipresent. While sight and sound can be blocked out of our awareness, the communications of touch never cease, announcing themselves in pleasure and pain, in breathing and movement, and even in the downward drag of my own organs under the force of gravity as I sit to write these words. Nothing else will suffice as a metaphor for the faithful, responsive closeness of God to each of us.

So to return to a question underlying this book, of "where is God in dementia?" the answer is, surely, that "the God who was physically incarnate as the body of Jesus Christ, who has never ceased to offer his body to us in the Sacraments and the community of the Church, in whose Glorified Body we will all be drawn together, in all our aspects and relationships, is right here: right here because he has never been away from us." We have been beguiled by our hypercognitive society, but the God who is to be found in dementia is incomparably bigger and closer than anything we can imagine as an extension of our shallow subjectivity. Here God is, with us *corps à corps*, closer than the very cells of our own bodies, everywhere and for ever. For who shall separate us from the love of Christ?

Bibliography

Alzheimer's Research UK. "Dementia Attitudes Monitor Wave 2." London, 2021.
———. "Rising to the Challenge: The Power to Defeat Dementia." London, 2014. https://www.alzheimersresearchuk.org/about-us/our-influence/policy-work/reports/defeat-dementia-report/.
Alzheimer's Society. "Alzheimer's Society CEO Responds to Criticism of Their Latest TV Campaign." 2024. https://www.alzheimers.org.uk/news/2024-3-24/ceo-responds-criticism.
———. "Caring for My Dad with Frontotemporal Dementia—Rachel's Story." Feb. 25, 2020. https://www.alzheimers.org.uk/blog/rachel-frontotemporal-dementia-ftd-story.
———. "The Long Goodbye: Our New Advert." 2024. https://www.alzheimers.org.uk/about-us/dementia-news-and-media/long-goodbye.
Anselm of Canterbury. *The Passion of Christ Through the Eyes of Mary*. Charlotte, NC: Tan, 2022.
Aquinas, Thomas. *The Summa Theologica: Complete Edition*. Edited by Fathers of the English Dominican Province. Oxford: Catholic Way, 2014.
Athanasius. *On the Incarnation*. Grand Rapids: Christian Classics Ethereal Library, n.d. https://ccel.org/ccel/athanasius/incarnation/incarnation.ix.html.
Atwell, Robert, et al. *God in Fragments: Worshipping with Those Living with Dementia*. London: Church House, 2020.
Aylwin, Michael. "'It Comes for Your Very Soul': How Alzheimer's Undid My Dazzling, Creative Wife in Her 40s." *The Guardian*, July 19, 2024. https://www.theguardian.com/news/article/2024/jul/09/how-alzheimers-undid-my-dazzling-creative-wife-in-her-40s.
Barclay, Aileen. "Lost in Eden: Dementia from Paradise." *Journal of Religion, Spirituality and Aging* 28.1–2 (2016) 68–83.
Baumgarten, Mona. "The Health of Persons Giving Care to the Demented Elderly: A Critical Review of the Literature." *Journal of Clinical Epidemiology* 42.12 (1989) 1137–48.
Baxley, Danny L., and Malcolm Goldsmith. "In a Strange Land . . . People with Dementia and the Local Church." *Dementia* 4.2 (2005) 317–19.
Behuniak, Susan M. "The Living Dead? The Construction of People with Alzheimer's Disease as Zombies." *Ageing and Society* 31.1 (2011) 70–92.
Berger, Peter L., and Thomas Luckmann. *The Social Construction of Reality: A Treatise in the Sociology of Knowledge*. New York: Doubleday, 1966.

Bibliography

Beuscher, Linda, and Cornelia Beck. "A Literature Review of Spirituality in Coping with Early-Stage Alzheimer's Disease." *Journal of Clinical Nursing* 17.5a (2008) 88–97.

Beuscher, Linda, and Victoria T. Grando. "Using Spirituality to Cope with Early-Stage Alzheimer's Disease." *Western Journal of Nursing Research* 31.5 (2009) 583–98.

Bohlmeijer, Ernst T., et al. "Narrative Foreclosure in Later Life: Preliminary Considerations for a New Sensitizing Concept." *Journal of Aging Studies* 25.4 (2011) 364–70.

Bonhoeffer, Dietrich. *Letters and Papers from Prison.* London: SCM, 2013.

Brock, Brian. *Wondrously Wounded: Theology, Disability and the Body of Christ.* Waco, TX: Baylor University Press, 2019.

Bryden, Christine. *Dancing with Dementia: My Story of Living Positively with Dementia.* London: Jessica Kingsley, 2005.

———. "A Spiritual Journey into the I–Thou Relationship: A Personal Reflection on Living with Dementia." *Journal of Religion, Spirituality and Aging* 28.1-2 (2016) 7–14.

———. *Who Will I Be When I Die?* London: Jessica Kingsley, 2012.

Bute, Jennifer. "Hello, My Name Is Jennifer Bute." Dementia Alliance International, 2022. https://dementiaallianceinternational.org/about/resources/our-voice-matters/hello-my-name-is-jennnifer-bute.

Bute, Jennifer, and Louise Morse. *Dementia from the Inside: A Doctor's Personal Journey of Hope.* London: SPCK, 2018.

Campbell, Alistair V. *Rediscovering Pastoral Care.* London: Darton, Longman and Todd, 1986.

Catholic Church. *Catechism of the Catholic Church.* New York: Bantam Doubleday, 1995.

Certeau, Michel de. *The Mystic Fable, Volume 1: The Sixteenth and Seventeenth Centuries.* Edited by Michael B. Smith. Chicago: University of Chicago Press, 1992.

Chapman, Michael, Jennifer Philip, and Paul Komesaroff. "A Person-Centred Problem." *Humanities and Social Sciences Communications* 9.1 (2022) 1–11.

Chauvet, Louis-Marie. *Symbol and Sacrament: A Sacramental Reinterpretation of Christian Existence.* Edited by Patrick Madigan and Madeleine Beaumont. Collegeville, MN: Liturgical, 1995.

Collicutt, Joanna. "Spiritual Awareness and Dementia." In *God in Fragments: Worshipping with Those Living with Dementia*, edited by Robert Atwell et al., 14–36. London: Church House, 2020.

———. *Thinking of You: A Resource for the Spiritual Care of People with Dementia.* Abingdon, UK: BRF, 2017.

Comensoli, Peter A. *In God's Image: Recognizing the Profoundly Impaired as Persons.* Eugene, OR: Cascade, 2018.

Cook, Christopher C. H. "The Lived Experience of Dementia: Developing a Contextual Theology." *Journal of Religion, Spirituality and Aging* 28.1-2 (2016) 84–97.

Crisp, Oliver D. *The Word Enfleshed: Exploring the Person and Work of Christ.* Ada, MI: Baker Academic, 2016.

Davis, Robert, and Betty Davis. *My Journey into Alzheimer's Disease.* Wheaton, IL: Tyndale House, 1989.

De Klerk-Rubin, Vicki, and Daniel C. Potts. "The Validation Method for Dementia Care." *Practical Neurology* (March/April 2022) 23–27.

De Lubac, Henri. *Corpus Mysticum: The Eucharist and the Church in the Middle Ages.* South Bend, IN: University of Notre Dame Press, 2007.

Bibliography

Descartes, Rene. *Discourse on Method*. [1637] Edited by F. E. Sutcliffe. London: Penguin Classics, 1968.
Douglas, Kelly Brown. *The Black Christ*. Vol. 9. Ossining, NY: Orbis, 2019.
Doyle, Kenneth. "Disruptions in Church." *The Pilot*, Oct. 13, 2021. https://www.thebostonpilot.com/AMP/amp_article.php?ID=190828.
Doyle, Patrick J., and Robert L. Rubinstein. "Person-Centered Dementia Care and the Cultural Matrix of Othering." *The Gerontologist* 54.6 (2013) 952–63.
Durkheim, Émile. *The Division of Labour in Society*. 1893. Edited by W. D. Halls. New York: Free Press, 1997.
Ehrman, Terrence. "Disability and Resurrection Identity." *New Blackfriars* 96.1066 (2015) 723–38.
Eiesland, Nancy L. *The Disabled God: Toward a Liberatory Theology of Disability*. Nashville: Abingdon, 1994.
Ekoh, P., et al. "An Appraisal of Public Understanding of Dementia Across Cultures." *Journal of Social Work in Developing Societies* 2.1 (2020) 54–67.
Ellor, James. "Celebrating the Human Spirit." In *God Never Forgets: Faith, Hope, and Alzheimer's Disease*, edited by Donald McKim, 1–20. Louisville, KY: Westminster John Knox, 1997.
Emery, Erin E., and Kenneth I. Pargament. "The Many Faces of Religious Coping in Late Life: Conceptualization, Measurement, and Links to Well-Being." *Ageing International* 29.1 (2004) 3–27.
Eriksen, Siren, et al. "The Experience of Lived Body as Expressed by People with Dementia: A Systematic Meta-Synthesis." *Dementia* 21.5 (2022) 1771–99.
Falque, Emmanuel. *La Chair de Dieu*. Paris: Cerf, 2023.
———. *Crossing the Rubicon: The Borderlands of Philosophy and Theology*. New York: Fordham University Press, 2016.
———. *God, the Flesh, and the Other: From Irenaeus to Duns Scotus*. Evanston, IL: Northwestern University Press, 2015.
———. *The Wedding Feast of the Lamb: Eros, the Body, and the Eucharist*. New York: Fordham University Press, 2016.
Fox, Judith. *I Still Do: Loving and Living with Alzheimer's*. New York: Powerhouse, 2009.
Fritzson, Arne. Review of *Vulnerable Communion* by Thomas Reynolds. *Ecumenical Review* 61.2 (2009) 241–43.
Fuchs, Thomas. "Embodiment and Personal Identity in Dementia." *Medicine, Health Care and Philosophy* 23.4 (2020) 665–76.
Fuchs, Thomas, Thiemo Breyer, and Christoph Mundt. *Karl Jaspers' Philosophy and Psychopathology*. Berlin: Springer, 2013.
Gabrielli, T. Review of *The Wedding Feast of the Lamb* by Emmanuel Falque. *Pray Tell* blog, 2018. https://praytellblog.com/index.php/2018/06/19/book-review-the-wedding-feast-of-the-lamb/.
Garrigou-Lagrange, Reginald. *The Three Ages of the Interior Life, Volumes 1 and 2*. Edited by M. Timothea Doyle. St. Louis: Herder, 1948.
George, Daniel R. "The Art of Medicine Overcoming the Social Death of Dementia Through Language." *The Lancet* 376.9741 (2010) 586–87.
Ghane, Golnar, et al. "Social Death in Patients: Concept Analysis with an Evolutionary Approach." *SSM–Population Health* 14 (2021) 100795.

Bibliography

Goldsmith, Malcolm. "Dementia: A Challenge to Christian Theology and Pastoral Care." In *Spirituality and Ageing*, edited by Albert Jewell, 125–35. London: Jessica Kingsley, 1999.

———. *Hearing the Voice of People with Dementia: Opportunities and Obstacles.* London: Jessica Kingsley, 1996.

Gosbell, Louise A. "Space, Place, and the Ordering of Materiality in Disability Theology: Locating Disability in the Resurrection and the Body of Christ." *Journal of Disability and Religion* 26.2 (2022) 149–61.

Greggs, Tom. "The Order and Movement of Eternity: Karl Barth on the Eternity of God and Creaturely Time." In *Eternal God, Eternal Life: Theological Investigations into the Concept of Immortality*, edited by Philip G. Zeigler, 1–24. London: Bloomsbury T&T Clark, 2018.

Gschwandtner, Christina M. "Corporeality, Animality, Bestiality: Emmanuel Falque on Incarnate Flesh." *Analecta Hermeneutica* 4 (2012) 1–16.

———. "Mystery Manifested: Toward a Phenomenology of the Eucharist in Its Liturgical Context." *Religions* 10.5 (2019) 315–32.

Habermas, Gary, Jonathan Kopel, and Benjamin C. F. Shaw. "Medical Views on the Death by Crucifixion of Jesus Christ." *Baylor University Medical Center Proceedings* 34.6 (2021) 748–52.

Harkaway-Krieger, Kerilyn. "Theology and Theories of Metaphor: How We Talk When We Talk About God." *Heythrop Journal* 65.4 (2024) 343–59.

Hauerwas, Stanley. *Suffering Presence: Theological Reflections on Medicine, the Mentally Handicapped and the Church.* Notre Dame, IN: University of Notre Dame 1988.

Hayes, Karen. "The Landscape of Dementia (Unpublished)." https://www.dementiapositive.co.uk/previous-quotations-of-the-month.html. Accessed July 29, 2024.

Hopkins, Denise Dombrowski. "Failing Brain, Faithful God." In *God Never Forgets: Faith, Hope, and Alzheimer's Disease*, edited by Donald McKim, 21–37. Louisville, KY: Westminster John Knox, 1997.

Horsburgh, Tamara. *The Impact of Holding Faith, Particularly the Christian Theologies of Hope and Suffering, When Diagnosed with Dementia: An IPA Study.* Paisley, UK: University of the West of Scotland, 2024.

Hudson, Rosalie Evelyn. "God's Faithfulness and Dementia: Christian Theology in Context." *Journal of Religion, Spirituality and Aging* 28.1–2 (2016) 50–67.

Hughes, Julian C. *Thinking Through Dementia.* Oxford: Oxford University Press, 2011.

Hughes, Julian C., Stephen J. Louw, and Steven R. Sabat, eds. *Dementia: Mind, Meaning, and the Person.* Oxford: Oxford University Press, 2006.

Hutchinson, Gloria. "Praying My Way Through Dementia." *St. Anthony Messenger.* Cincinnati, March 2020. https://www.franciscanmedia.org/st-anthony-messenger/march-2020/praying-my-way-through-dementia/.

Irenaeus. *Against Heresies.* Ante-Nicene Fathers, Vol. 1. Edited by Alexander Roberts. Reprint, Eugene, OR: Wipf & Stock, 2022.

Isherwood, Lisa. *The Fat Jesus: Christianity and Body Image.* New York: Church Publishing, 2008.

James, Rob, and Becca Stevens. "Behold, the Human Being: Hans Urs von Balthasar's Theology of the Paschal Triduum and the Self in Dementia." *Theology* 126.2 (2023) 103–10.

Bibliography

Janicaud, Dominique. "The Theological Turn of French Phenomenology." In *Phenomenology and the "Theological Turn": The French Debate*, 3–103. New York: Fordham University Press, 2000.

Jaynes, Julian. *The Origin of Consciousness in the Breakdown of the Bicameral Mind*. Boston: Mariner, 2000.

Joh, Wonhee Anne. *Heart of the Cross: A Postcolonial Christology*. Louisville, KY: Presbyterian, 2006.

Johnstone, Megan-Jane. *Alzheimer's Disease, Media Representations and the Politics of Euthanasia: Constructing Risk and Selling Death in an Ageing Society*. London: Routledge, 2016.

———. "Metaphors, Stigma and the 'Alzheimerization' of the Euthanasia Debate." *Dementia* 12.4 (2013) 377–93.

Keck, David. *Forgetting Whose We Are*. Nashville: Abingdon, 1996.

Kevern, Peter. "The Grace of Foolishness: What Christians with Dementia Can Bring to the Churches." *Practical Theology* 2.2 (2009) 205–18.

———. "'I Pray That I Will Not Fall over the Edge.' What Is Left of Faith After Dementia?" *Practical Theology* 4.3 (2011) 283–94.

———. "Sharing the Mind of Christ: Preliminary Thoughts on Dementia and the Cross." *New Blackfriars* 91.1034 (2010) 408–22.

———. "Spirituality and Dementia." In *The Routledge International Handbook of Spirituality in Society and the Professions*, edited by Laszlo Zsolnai and Bernadette Flanagan, 223–30. London: Routledge, 2019.

———. "The Spirituality of People with Late-Stage Dementia: A Review of the Research Literature, a Critical Analysis and Some Implications for Person-Centred Spirituality and Dementia Care." *Mental Health, Religion and Culture* 18.9 (2015) 765–76.

———. "What Sort of a God Is to Be Found in Dementia? A Survey of Theological Responses and an Agenda for Their Development." *Theology* 113.873 (2010) 174–82.

Kevern, Peter, and David Primrose. "Changes in Measures of Dementia Awareness in UK Church Congregations Following a 'Dementia-Friendly' Intervention: A Pre–Post Cohort Study." *Religions* 11.7 (2020) 337–48.

Kiblinger, Kristin. "Theology of Dementia and Caputo's 'Difficult Glory.'" *Journal of Disability and Religion* 28.2 (2023) 148–63.

Killick, John. *Poetry and Dementia: A Practical Guide*. London: Jessica Kingsley, 2017.

———. *You Are Words: Dementia Poems*. London: Journal of Dementia Care, 2008.

Killick, John, and Carl Cordonnier. *Openings: Dementia Poems and Photographs*. London: Hawker, 2000.

Kilner, John F. *Dignity and Destiny: Humanity in the Image of God*. Grand Rapids: Eerdmans, 2015.

Kim, Jiyoung, and Nayeon Shin. "Development of the 'Living Well' Concept for Older People with Dementia." *BMC Geriatrics* 23.1 (2023) 611–22.

Kitwood, T. *Dementia Reconsidered: The Person Comes First*. Milton Keynes, UK: Open University, 1997.

Kontos, Pia, and Wendy Martin. "Embodiment and Dementia: Exploring Critical Narratives of Selfhood, Surveillance, and Dementia Care." *Dementia* 12.3 (2013) 288–302.

Krueger, Derek. "From Comedy to Martyrdom: The Shifting Theology of the Holy Fool from Symeon of Emesa to Andres." In *Holy Fools and Divine Madmen: Sacred Insanity Through Ages and Cultures*, edited by Albrecht Berger and Sergey Ivanov,

Bibliography

29–48. Munich: Ars una, 2018. http://www.escholarship.org/editions/view?docId=ft6k4007sx;brand=eschol.

———. *Symeon the Holy Fool: Leontius's Life and the Late Antique City*. Transformation of the Classical Heritage 25. Berkeley: University of California, 1996.

Linthicum, Dorothy, and Janice Hicks. *Redeeming Dementia: Spirituality, Theology, and Science*. New York: Church, 2018.

Low, Lee-fay, and Farah Purwaningrum. "Negative Stereotypes, Fear and Social Distance: A Systematic Review of Depictions of Dementia in Popular Culture in the Context of Stigma." *BMC Geriatrics* 20 (2020) 1–16.

MacKinlay, Elizabeth. "Journeys with People Who Have Dementia: Connecting and Finding Meaning in the Journey." *Journal of Religion, Spirituality and Aging* 28.1–2 (2016) 24–36.

MacKinlay, Shane. "Eyes Wide Shut: A Response to Jean-Luc Marion's Account of the Journey to Emmaus." *Modern Theology* 20.3 (2004) 447–56.

Marion, Jean-Luc. *Being Given: Toward a Phenomenology of Givenness*. Redwood, CA: Stanford University Press, 2002.

———. *Believing in Order to See: On the Rationality of Revelation and the Irrationality of Some Believers*. New York: Fordham University Press, 2017.

———. "The Saturated Phenomenon." *Philosophy Today* 40.1 (1996) 103–24.

Martin, Dale B. *The Corinthian Body*. New Haven, CT: Yale University Press, 1995.

Mason, Clare, et al. "Language About People with Dementia." In *A Critical History of Dementia Studies*, edited by James Fletcher and Andrea Capstick, 41–54. London: Routledge, 2024.

Mast, Benjamin T. *Second Forgetting: Remembering the Power of the Gospel During Alzheimer's Disease*. Grand Rapids: Zondervan, 2014.

McFarland, Ian. *The Divine Image: Envisioning the Invisible God*. Philadelphia: Fortress, 2005.

McGrath, Alister E. *Historical Theology: An Introduction to the History of Christian Thought*. 2nd ed. Oxford: Wiley-Blackwell, 2013.

McKim, Donald K., ed. *God Never Forgets: Faith, Hope, and Alzheimer's Disease*. Louisville, KY: Westminster John Knox, 1997.

Meeting Centres UK. "The Evidence Behind Meeting Centres." Worcester, UK: University of Worcester, 2022.

Mitchell, Wendy. "My Final Hug in a Mug . . . ." *Which Me Am I Today?* blog, Feb. 12, 2024. https://whichmeamitoday.wordpress.com/blog/.

Moltmann, Jürgen. *The Crucified God*. London: SCM, 1974.

Moltmann-Wendel, Elisabeth. "Is There a Feminist Theology of the Cross?" In *The Scandal of a Crucified World*, edited by Y. Tesfai, 87–98. New York: Orbis, 1994.

Morse, Louise, and Roger Hitchings. *Could It Be Dementia? Losing Your Mind Doesn't Mean Losing Your Soul*. Oxford: Monarch, 2008.

Naue, Ursula, and Thilo Kroll. "'The Demented Other': Identity and Difference in Dementia." *Nursing Philosophy* 10 (2009) 26–33.

Oakes, Edward T. "The Internal Logic of Holy Saturday in the Theology of Hans Urs von Balthasar." *International Journal of Systematic Theology* 9.2 (2007) 184–99.

Ogude, James. *Ubuntu and Personhood*. Trenton, NJ: Africa World Press, 2018.

Pappas, Jack Louis. "Between the Flesh and the Lived Body." *Journal for Continental Philosophy of Religion* 2.1 (2020) 73–90.

Bibliography

Pope Francis. "General Audience." Rome, March 11, 2015. https://www.vatican.va/content/francesco/en/audiences/2015/documents/papa-francesco_20150311_udienza-generale.html.

Pope Paul VI. *Lumen Gentium*. Rome, November 21, 1964. https://www.vatican.va/archive/hist_councils/ii_vatican_council/documents/vat-ii_const_19641121_lumen-gentium_en.html.

———. *Sacrosanctum Concilium*. Rome, December 4, 1963. https://www.vatican.va/archive/hist_councils/ii_vatican_council/documents/vat-ii_const_19631204_sacrosanctum-concilium_en.html#.

Pope Pius XII. *Mystici Corporis Christi*. Rome, June 29, 1943. https://www.vatican.va/content/pius-xii/en/encyclicals/documents/hf_p-xii_enc_29061943_mystici-corporis-christi.html.

Post, Stephen. "The Concept of Alzheimer Disease in a Hypercognitive Society." In *Concepts of Alzheimer Disease: Biological, Clinical and Cultural Perspectives*, edited by Jesse F. Ballenger, Konrad Maurer and Peter J. Whitehouse, 245–56. Baltimore: Johns Hopkins University Press, 2000.

———. *The Moral Challenge of Alzheimer Disease: Ethical Issues from Diagnosis to Dying*. Baltimore: Johns Hopkins University Press, 2002.

———. "Respectare: Moral Respect for the Lives of the Deeply Forgetful." In *Dementia: Mind, Meaning and the Person*, edited by Julian C. Hughes, Stephen J. Louw, and Steven R. Sabat, 223–34. Oxford: Oxford University Press, 2006.

Poulakou-Rebelakou, E., et al. "Holy Fools: A Religious Phenomenon of Extreme Behaviour." *Journal of Religion and Health* 53.1 (2014) 95–104.

Radden, J., and J. Fordyce. "Into the Darkness: Losing Identity with Dementia." In *Dementia: Mind, Meaning and the Person*, edited by Julian C. Hughes, Stephen J. Louw, and Steven R. Sabat, 71–88. Oxford: Oxford University Press, 2006.

Reinders, Hans S. *Receiving the Gift of Friendship: Profound Disability, Theological Anthropology, and Ethics*. Grand Rapids: Eerdmans, 2008.

Reynolds, Thomas E. *Vulnerable Communion: A Theology of Disability and Hospitality*. Ada, MI: Brazos, 2008.

Ricoeur, Paul. *Interpretation Theory: Discourse and the Surplus of Meaning*. Fort Worth, TX: Texas Christian University Press, 1976.

Rohr, Richard. *Immortal Diamond: The Search for Our True Self*. New York: Wiley & Sons, 2012.

Rosenbaum, Ron. "Elie Wiesel's Secret." *Tablet*, Sept. 28, 2017. https://www.tabletmag.com/sections/arts-letters/articles/elie-wiesels-secret.

Ruin, Hans. "Saying the Sacred: Notes Towards a Phenomenology of Prayer." In *Phenomenology and Religion: New Frontiers*, edited by Jonna Bornemark and Hans Ruin, högskola Södertörn, 291–309. Huddinge: Södertörn University Press, 2010.

Sabat, Steven R. *The Experience of Alzheimer's Disease: Life Through a Tangled Veil*. Hoboken, NJ: Wiley-Blackwell, 2001.

Sabat, Steven R., et al. "The 'Demented Other' or Simply 'a Person'? Extending the Philosophical Discourse of Naue and Kroll Through the Situated Self." *Nursing Philosophy* 12.4 (2011) 282–92.

Sacks, Oliver. *The Man Who Mistook His Wife for a Hat: And Other Clinical Tales*. New York: Simon and Schuster, 1998.

Bibliography

Saliers, Don E. "Toward a Spirituality of Inclusiveness." In *Human Disability and the Service of God: Reassessing Religious Practice*, edited by Nancy Eiesland and Don Saliers, 19–31. Nashville: Abingdon, 1998.

Sapp, Stephen. "Memory: The Community Looks Backward." In *God Never Forgets: Faith, Hope and Alzheimer's Disease*, edited by Donald McKim, 38–54. Louisville, KY: Westminster John Knox, 1997.

Saward, John. *Perfect Fools: Folly for Christ's Sake in Catholic and Orthodox Spirituality*. Oxford: Oxford University Press, 1980.

Scarry, Elaine. *The Body in Pain: The Making and Unmaking of the World*. Oxford: Oxford University Press, 1988.

Schlingheider, Regina. "The Eucharist, Dementia, and Time." *Journal of Religion, Spirituality and Aging* 36.2 (2024) 173–87.

Scott, Roger. Review of *Symeon the Holy Fool: Leontius's Life and the Late Antique City* by Derek Krueger. *Transformation* 3.7 (1997). https://scholar.lib.vt.edu/ejournals/ElAnt/V3N7/scott.html.

Shabahangi, N. R. "Redefining Dementia: Between the World of Forgetting and Remembering." Personal communication, 2005.

Shepheard, Amanda, and Lauren Woodrow. "GPs to Bear the Brunt of Dementia 'Tsunami.'" *The Medical Republic*, Feb. 22, 2024. https://www.medicalrepublic.com.au/gps-to-bear-the-brunt-of-dementia-tsunami/105393.

Simango, Daniel. "The Imago Dei (Gen 1:26–27): A History of Interpretation from Philo to the Present." *Studia Historiae Ecclesiasticae* 42.1 (2016) 172–90.

Simpson, Julie. *"I Still, I Still, I Still, I Still . . . ." The Voice of the Older Person with Advanced Dementia in Residential Aged Care: An Ethnography Exploring What It Means for the Person to Have Their Voice*. Adelaide: Flinders University, 2024.

Sloane, Andrew. "The Dissolving Self? Dementia and Identity in Philosophical Theology." *Science and Christian Belief* 31.2 (2019) 131–51.

Snyder, Lisa. "Satisfactions and Challenges in Spiritual Faith and Practice for Persons with Dementia." *Dementia: The International Journal of Social Research and Practice*, Spirituality and Dementia, 2.3 (2003) 299–313.

Sonderegger, Katherine. "Towards a Doctrine of Resurrection." In *Eternal God, Eternal Life: Theological Investigations into the Concept of Immortality*, edited by Philip G. Zeigler, 115–30. London: Bloomsbury T&T Clark, 2018.

Spitzer, Robert J. "The Stages of Christian Mysticism—a Summary." May 2016. https://7693347.fs1.hubspotusercontent-na1.net/hubfs/7693347/MC_Spitzer%20Scholarly%20Articles/Christian-Mysticism.pdf.

Sweeting, Helen, and Mary Gilhooly. "Dementia and the Phenomenon of Social Death." *Sociology of Health and Illness* 19.1 (1997) 93–117.

Swinton, John. *Becoming Friends of Time: Disability, Timefullness, and Gentle Discipleship*. London: SCM, 2017.

———. *Dementia: Living in the Memories of God*. London: SCM, 2012.

———. "Remembering the Person: Theological Reflections on God, Personhood and Dementia." In *Ageing, Disability and Spirituality*, edited by Elizabeth MacKinlay, 22–35. London: Jessica Kingsley, 2008.

Teilhard de Chardin, Pierre. *Le Milieu Divin*. London: Fontana, 1964.

Thornton, Timothy. "The Discursive Turn, Social Constructionism, and Dementia." In *Dementia: Mind, Meaning, and the Person*, edited by Julian C. Hughes, Stephen J. Louw, and Steven R. Sabat, 125–41. Oxford: Oxford University Press, 2006.

Bibliography

Ticciati, Susannah. "Resurrection of the Dead." *St. Andrews Encyclopaedia of Theology.* Online, 2023. https://www.saet.ac.uk/Christianity/ResurrectionoftheDead.

Tillich, Paul. *Systematic Theology, Volume I.* Chicago: University of Chicago Press, 1951.

Treanor, David P. *Intellectual Disability and Social Policies of Inclusion: Invading Consciousness Without Permeability.* Berlin: Springer Nature, 2020.

Trevitt, Corinne, and Elizabeth MacKinlay. "'Just Because I Can't Remember . . . .' Religiousness in Older People with Dementia." In *Spirituality of Later Life*, edited by Elizabeth MacKinlay, 109–21. London: Routledge, 2014.

UsAgainstAlzheimer's. "The Alzheimer's Disease Crisis—By the Numbers." 2024. https://www.usagainstalzheimers.org/learn/alzheimers-crisis.

Vance, David E., et al. "Practical Implications of Procedural and Emotional Religious Activity Therapy for Nursing." *Journal of Gerontological Nursing* 36.8 (2010) 22–29.

Van De Creek, Larry. *Spiritual Care for Persons with Dementia: Fundamentals for Pastoral Practice.* Abingdon, UK: Routledge, 2015.

Vanstone, W. H. *The Stature of Waiting.* London: Darton, Longman and Todd, 1982.

Waddell, Michael M. "Thomas Aquinas and the Resurrection of the (Disabled) Body." *The Saint Anselm Journal* 12.1 (2017) 29–51.

Ware, Kallistos. "'In the Image and Likeness': The Uniqueness of the Human Person." In *Theological Anthropology, 500 Years After Martin Luther*, edited by Christophe Chalamet et al., 48–64. Leiden: Brill, 2021.

Watson, Rochelle, et al. "Dementia Is the Second Most Feared Condition Among Australian Health Service Consumers: Results of a Cross-Sectional Survey." *BMC Public Health* 23.1 (2023) 1–7.

Watts, Fraser. *A Plea for Embodied Spirituality: The Role of the Body in Religion.* Eugene, OR: Wipf & Stock, 2022.

Weinandy, Thomas. *Does God Suffer?* South Bend, IN: University of Notre Dame Press, 2000.

Whitaker, Maja I. "Perfected yet Still Disabled? Continuity of Embodied Identity in Resurrection Life." *Stimulus: The New Zealand Journal of Christian Thought and Practice* 26.2 (2019) 18–25.

Widdershoven, Guy A. M., and Ron L. P. Berghmans. "Meaning-Making in Dementia: A Hermeneutic Perspective." In *Dementia: Mind, Meaning, and the Person*, edited by Julian C. Hughes, Stephen J. Louw, and Steven R. Sabat, 179–91. Oxford: Oxford University Press, 2006.

Williams, Patricia. *God's Not Forgotten Me: Experiencing Faith in Dementia.* Eugene, OR: Cascade, 2022.

———. "Knowing God in Dementia: What Happens to Faith When You Can No Longer Remember?" *Health and Social Care Chaplaincy* 4.2 (2016) 142–57.

———. *What Happens to Faith When Christians Get Dementia? The Faith Experience and Practice of Evangelical Christians Living with Mild to Moderate Dementia.* Eugene, OR: Pickwick, 2021.

Williams, Thomas D., and Jan Olof Bengtsson. "Personalism." *Stanford Encyclopedia of Philosophy*, 2009. https://plato.stanford.edu/entries/personalism/.

Wilson, Clare. "What Dementia 'Tsunami'? Your Chances of Getting It Have Dropped." *New Scientist*, Aug. 21, 2015. https://www.newscientist.com/article/dn28079-what-dementia-tsunami-your-chances-of-getting-it-have-dropped/.

World Health Organization. "Dementia." Health Topics Fact Sheets, 2023. https://www.who.int/news-room/fact-sheets/detail/dementia.

Bibliography

Yong, Amos. *The Bible, Disability, and the Church: A New Vision of the People of God*. Grand Rapids: Eerdmans, 2011.

———. "Disability, the Human Condition, and the Spirit of the Eschatological Long Run: Toward a Pneumatological Theology of Disability." *Journal of Religion, Disability and Health* 11.1 (2007) 5–25.

———. *Theology and Down Syndrome: Reimagining Disability in Late Modernity*. Waco, TX: Baylor University Press, 2007.

Zeigler, Philip G. "Editor's Introduction." In *Eternal God, Eternal Life: Theological Investigations into the Concept of Immortality*, edited by Philip G. Zeigler, vii–xii. London: T&T Clark, 2016.

www.ingramcontent.com/pod-product-compliance
Lightning Source LLC
Chambersburg PA
CBHW030858170426
43193CB00009BA/651